YOGA: Complete Guide to Slimming at Home with the Chair.

Practical yoga manual with simple exercises to do at home. Uses chair and home tools for a slimming and effective application program.

By Francesco Martini

A GIFT FOR YOU!

Dear reader,

Thank you for choosing to purchase YOGA: Complete Guide to Slimming at Home with the Chair! To express my gratitude, I've decided to offer you an exclusive gift:

10 YOGA FACIAL EXERCISES.

Discover the effectiveness of facial yoga with this exclusive ebook! You'll find 10 targeted exercises to tone, firm and relax facial muscles, stimulating circulation and visibly reducing signs of fatigue and aging. A simple and natural routine for a fresh, radiant and youthful face.

To access your free and exclusive gift, simply scan this QR code:

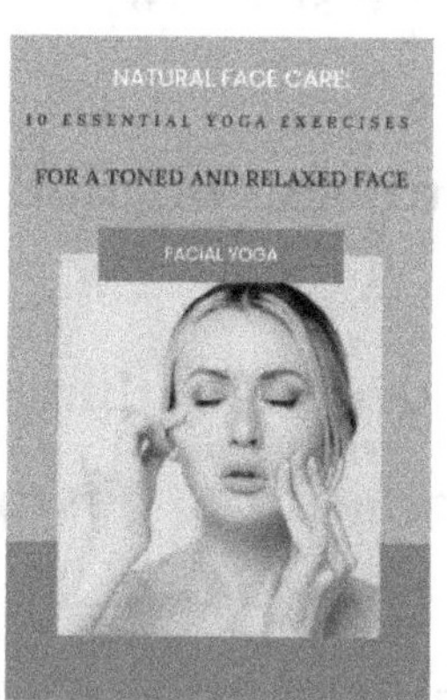

I hope this gift adds even more value to your reading experience and helps you achieve your goals. Enjoy your reading and thank you once again for your support!

Chapter 1: Introduction to Yoga for Weight Loss

1.1 What is yoga and why it helps you lose weight

Yoga is an ancient practice that combines movement, breathing and meditation to create balance between body and mind. But in addition to its well-known mental and spiritual benefits, yoga can also be a powerful tool for weight loss. Unlike cardio or weight-bearing exercises, yoga works in a more gentle but equally effective way, stimulating the body on a physical and metabolic level.

Why does yoga help with weight loss? The answer lies in the way this discipline works on several fronts. First, many of the yoga postures, called *asanas*, require strength and endurance. These postures engage muscles in a profound way, activating both major and stabilizing muscles that are often not stimulated by other types of exercise. Even postures that look static require constant work to maintain balance, toning and strengthening the body.

In addition, yoga improves metabolism. Dynamic sequences, such as *Vinyasa* or *Surya Namaskar* (Sun Salutation), create a flow of movement that speeds up the heart rate and increases calorie burning, similar to light aerobic activity. Although the pace is not as fast as a run or a high-intensity workout, the body continues to burn calories more consistently and prolonged, even after practice.

Another key aspect of slimming through yoga is stress management. Excess stress is often linked to weight gain, especially in the abdominal area, due to high cortisol production. Yoga, with its focus on deep breathing and meditation, helps reduce cortisol levels in the body, thus improving the ability to lose weight. When the mind is calm and relaxed, food choices also become more mindful, reducing emotional binge eating or stress eating.

Finally, yoga promotes body awareness. During practice, we learn to tune in to our body's signals, better understanding when we are hungry or thirsty, and what makes us feel better. This leads to a healthier and more intuitive approach toward nutrition, which is essential to achieving and maintaining lasting results in weight loss.

1.2 <u>Specific benefits of doing yoga at home</u>

Choosing to do yoga in the comfort of your own home offers many advantages, allowing anyone to practice flexibly, without constraints of time or place. One of the main strengths is the freedom to tailor sessions to your needs, without having to adhere to strict schedules or reach a specific center. You can decide when and how to practice, integrating yoga into your daily routine with great ease.

Creating a customized environment for practice is another positive aspect: you can make the space relaxing and welcoming by choosing the right music, adjusting the lighting, and preparing everything you need. This level of customization facilitates a deeper connection with yourself, fostering a more intimate and focused experience. Without external distractions, such as the dynamics of a group or the rhythms of a group class, it becomes easier to maintain focus on breath and movement.

One of the main advantages is the ability to practice consistently, even if you have little time. You can fit short yoga sessions into your day, taking advantage of as little as 15 or 20 minutes to relax your mind and work on your body. You don't need to have long hours; a short, regular practice can still lead to significant improvements in muscle tone, flexibility, and mental well-being. This daily approach is easier to maintain when there is no commute or set schedule to keep.

Another important aspect is the ability to practice at your own pace, without feeling obligated to follow the level of a group. You can leisurely explore the positions, delve into the ones you find most useful, and give yourself the time you need to improve. This makes the home environment perfect both for beginners, who can take their time to learn, and for those who want a more relaxed and personalized practice.

Finally, practicing yoga at home is cheap and simple. No special equipment is needed-a chair, mat, or a few household items are more than enough. This makes yoga accessible to everyone, eliminating additional costs and making it easier to incorporate the practice into everyday life.

1.3 <u>The importance of constancy and breathing</u>

Consistency is one of the key elements in achieving lasting results in yoga practice, especially when the goal is weight loss. A regular practice, even if brief, is much more effective than intense but sporadic sessions. In fact, yoga works progressively on the body and mind, fostering gradual improvements that, over time, are consolidated. Maintaining a consistent routine allows you to strengthen muscles, improve flexibility and, crucially, stimulate metabolism, which is an essential factor in weight loss.

Creating a daily habit, even of only 15-20 minutes, allows the body to gradually adapt to the efforts and stimuli of practice. With consistency, one develops not only physical strength, but also greater awareness of oneself and one's body. This process, over time, helps to refine postures, improve balance and increase the effectiveness of the exercises. In addition, regular practice helps keep the mind focused, improving the ability to relax and reduce stress, a factor often linked to weight gain.

Another crucial aspect of yoga is breathing, known as Pranayama. Breathing correctly not only helps maintain calmness and concentration during practice, but directly affects the ability to burn calories and improve overall health. Deep, mindful breathing oxygenates the body optimally, promoting greater physical endurance and improved metabolism. In addition, well-controlled breathing helps reduce levels of the stress hormone cortisol, which, when elevated, can hinder weight loss.

In many postures, breathing plays a key role in stretching and holding. Inhaling deeply allows the muscles to expand, while exhaling helps them relax and enter the posture more easily. This continuous cycle of breathing, coordinated with movement, creates a smooth and harmonious practice that promotes not only physical but also mental well-being.

Being consistent in practice and breath management is therefore the key to getting the most out of yoga. There is no need to seek perfection in the postures right away, but rather to cultivate patience and determination in repeating the exercises regularly, letting your breathing guide each movement. In this way, the benefits will not be long in coming, making the path to weight loss smoother and more natural.

1.4 <u>Use of household tools such as the chair</u>

The chair, a common object in every home, can turn into an extremely useful tool for yoga practice. It is often thought that special equipment or dedicated environments are needed to do yoga, but in reality, everyday items such as a simple chair can offer crucial support, especially for those who are new to yoga or have difficulty performing the positions on the floor.

The use of the chair in yoga allows many of the traditional postures to be adapted, making them more accessible and safe. For example, balancing postures such as *Vrksasana* (tree) can be performed with chair support to stabilize the body and maintain balance, reducing the risk of falls. This is especially useful for those with limited mobility or those who want to improve balance without overstretching their muscles.

Stretching and flexibility postures can also be modified with the help of the chair. For example, *Uttanasana* (forward bending) can be performed with the hands resting on the backrest, allowing the back and legs to be stretched without having to reach down to the floor. In this way, anyone can benefit from stretching without putting undue pressure on muscles not yet ready for more advanced positions. This approach helps prevent injury, making the practice more sustainable over time.

In addition, the chair is particularly useful for core, leg and gluteal toning exercises. Positions such as planks or lunges can be adapted to use the chair as a support point. This not only makes it easier to perform the exercises, but also makes it possible to maintain proper posture and alignment, an essential factor in working the muscles effectively and safely. By using the chair as a support, controlled and concentrated movements can be performed, optimizing effort and reducing the risk of posture errors.

Finally, chair yoga is also a perfect practice for those who want to do quick and easy exercises throughout the day, perhaps during a work break or in a moment of relaxation. You don't need a lot of space or time-the chair becomes your portable yoga mat, always available for you to stretch, relax, and strengthen your body at any time.

Taking advantage of household tools, such as a chair, makes yoga more accessible, allowing anyone to benefit from the practice, regardless of experience level or physical limitations.

1.5 Introduction to the positive mindset for slimming

One of the most important aspects of achieving lasting results in slimming through yoga is developing a positive mindset. While exercise and a balanced diet play a key role, the mindset with which you approach the journey is equally decisive. Often, weight-loss-related failures stem from unrealistic expectations or a negative view of self. For this reason, it is essential to cultivate a mindset that is supportive and motivating, so that you approach the process with confidence and patience.

Positive mindset is not just about thinking optimistically, but rather about recognizing the value of the path itself. Every small step is progress, and yoga, with its focus on mindfulness, can help you develop this view. Daily practice teaches you to be present, to focus on what your body is doing at that moment, without worrying about immediate results. Over time, this attitude will enable you to welcome the changes taking place in your body with serenity, without judgment or frustration.

Another crucial aspect is patience. Weight loss does not happen overnight, and keeping a positive mindset means being able to accept this fact. Instead of focusing on the pounds lost, focus on the overall well-being you are building: more energy, more strength, more balance. Learn to enjoy every progress, no matter how small it may seem.

To support this mindset, repetition of positive affirmations is an excellent tool. Affirmations help you refocus your mind toward constructive and motivating thoughts, which facilitate the process of physical change. Below are 10 phrases to repeat every day to support your weight loss journey with a positive mindset:

1. **I welcome each step of my journey with patience and gratitude.**

2. **My body is strong and capable of transformation.**

3. **I take care of myself, one day at a time.**

4. **Every exercise I do brings me closer to my goal.**

5. **I am grateful for the strength and energy I am building.**

6. **Change starts from the inside and is reflected on the outside.**

7. **I feel better and fitter with each passing day.**

8. **Respecting my body means listening to it and nurturing it with love.**

9. **I am constant in my practice and I see the results.**

10. **I focus on progress, not perfection.**

Repeating these affirmations every day can help you maintain focus, turning your attitude toward losing weight into a positive and motivating experience. With a strong and confident mindset, accompanied by the practice of yoga, your journey will be not only effective but also rewarding.

Chapter 2: Preparing for Yoga Practice at Home

2.1 How to create a serene yoga space at home

Creating a dedicated space for yoga practice is essential to promote concentration and relaxation, making each session more effective and enjoyable. You don't need a lot of space or expensive equipment, but it is important to arrange an environment that is quiet, comfortable and free of distractions, so as to facilitate connection with your body and mind.

To begin, choose a corner of the house where you feel comfortable and that you can easily turn into your yoga space. This can be a corner of the living room, bedroom or even a small balcony. The important thing is that there is enough space for you to stretch out comfortably and perform the postures unobstructed. If possible, choose a place near a window to take advantage of the natural light that helps create a serene and rejuvenating atmosphere.

In terms of equipment, there is no need to invest a lot of money. The basic tools for a home practice are affordable and easy to find. Here are some essentials and where to find them:

- **Yoga mat**: This is the main tool. Choose a mat that is non-slip and comfortable to protect your joints during floor positions. You can find good quality cheap mats in stores such as Decathlon or on Amazon, with prices starting at about 10-15 euros.

- **Yoga pillow or blocks**: Although not essential, these accessories help you adjust positions and improve comfort. If you want to save money, you can use a pillow or folded towel for support. Cheap yoga blocks are easily found online or in sports stores for less than 10 euros.

- **Strap or elastic band**: Used to facilitate stretches and improve flexibility. Again, an inexpensive solution may be a simple belt or scarf, which can do the same job as a yoga-specific strap.

- **Stable** chair: A chair with a backrest, preferably without armrests, will be useful for supported positions. No need to buy a new one: just use a sturdy chair you already own.

To create a relaxing atmosphere, you can add a personal touch with a scented candle, incense, or a soft light lamp, all of which can be found at low prices in stores such as IKEA or Tiger. The important thing is that the space reflects your personality and makes you feel at peace. With these small touches and a low budget, you will have a cozy and functional yoga space in your home, ready to welcome your daily practice.

2.2 The importance of timing and clothing choice

One of the key aspects of an effective yoga practice is choosing the right time of day to practice. Each person has different rhythms, so it is important to find a time that suits your needs and allows you to focus fully. In general, many practitioners find it helpful to do yoga early in the morning, as the mind is fresh and the body can benefit from a gentle and progressive awakening. Morning practice helps set the tone for the day, fostering a sense of energy and inner calm that will stay with you well into the evening.

If mornings don't suit your lifestyle, you can choose to practice in the late afternoon or evening as a way to relax and let go of stress accumulated during the day. The important thing is to be consistent: even just 15 to 20 minutes of practice a day can make a big difference in improving flexibility, strength, and mental well-being. Find a time when you know you can be quiet and uninterrupted, making it part of your daily routine.

Choice of clothing for yoga practice

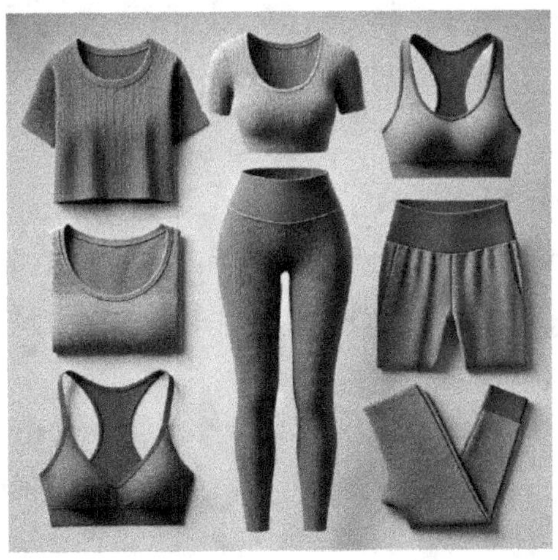

When choosing clothing to do yoga, it is essential to aim for garments that are comfortable, breathable and allow total freedom of movement. Here's what I recommend:

- **Yoga pants**: Choose stretchy, close-fitting pants, preferably high-waisted to ensure support and comfort during different postures. The ideal material is stretch cotton or technical spandex fabric, which offers flexibility and breathability. These pants are ideal for postures that require mobility and stability.

- **Shirt or top**: Opt for a tight-fitting shirt, such as a tank top or fitted T-shirt, made of a technical fabric that absorbs sweat and keeps the body dry during practice. Again, it is important that the fabric is stretchy and not too loose, to prevent it from impeding movement.

You can find these garments in sporting goods stores like **Decathlon**, which offers great garments at affordable prices, or on online platforms like **Amazon**. Look for brands like **Domyos** or **IUGA** for quality and affordability.

2.3 Equipment needed: chair, blankets, pillows

Although yoga does not require special equipment, some simple and readily available tools at home can make your practice safer, more comfortable and effective. Using common objects such as a chair, blankets and pillows will help you perform the postures correctly, easing muscle work and protecting joints.

The chair

A chair is one of the most versatile tools for yoga, ideal for those who have difficulty practicing on the floor or for those who want support during challenging postures. A sturdy chair, preferably without armrests, will help you perform balancing postures, such as Tree (*Vrksasana*), or bending postures, such as Forward Bend (*Uttanasana*). It will also be useful for toning exercises, such as lunges and modified planks, where the chair provides a foothold to make the exercises more accessible and safe.

Blankets Blankets can be used in a variety of ways to enhance your practice. Folded below the knees, they provide extra cushioning in postures that require you to be on the floor, such as the Downward Dog Posture (*Adho Mukha Svanasana*) or the Child's Posture *(Balasana)*. In addition, they can be useful during seated postures to raise the pelvis slightly, promoting correct posture and improving alignment of the spine. Blankets can also be used during the final relaxation, to cover oneself and keep the body warm and relaxed.

Pillows

Pillows, or a bolster (yoga-specific pillow), are good for providing support in relaxation and stretching postures. In the twisting or chest-opening postures, such as the Reclining Goddess Posture (*Supta Baddha Konasana*), a pillow under the back or between the legs can make it easier to maintain posture without undue strain. Even in seated postures, a pillow under the pelvis helps improve stability and reduce tension in the hips.

These simple tools found in every home can transform your practice, making it more comfortable and accessible, allowing you to adapt each position to your physical needs.

2.4 Tips for a relaxing environment

Creating a relaxing environment is critical to fostering a deep yoga practice, not only on a physical level, but also on a mental level. A well-organized, serene and distraction-free space will allow you to focus better and get the maximum benefit from your practice. Here I will explain how to set up your yoga space in a way that creates an atmosphere of calm and well-being, using simple but effective elements.

Lighting Adequate lighting is essential to create a relaxing environment. I recommend using warm, soft lights, such as lamps with light fabric shades or electric candles, which cast a soft light. Avoid lights that are too bright or cold, which can disrupt concentration. If you have a window, take advantage of natural light, which is perfect for morning sessions. Turn on dim lights before you begin your evening practice, so you can create a gentle transition to a relaxing atmosphere. You can find dimmable lamps or electric candles at stores like **IKEA** or online at **Amazon**, with a wide selection of inexpensive products.

Scents
Another key element for a relaxing environment is scent. Aromatherapy can help you enter a state of tranquility and concentration. Light an essential

oil diffuser or incense before your practice. Essential oils such as lavender, eucalyptus, or sandalwood are ideal for promoting relaxation. Use a small diffuser that does not invade the space and place it in a corner of the room. Electric diffusers and essential oils can be purchased at herbalists, home improvement stores, or on **Amazon**.

Music

A playlist with nature sounds or low volume ambient music can promote mental relaxation. Choose gentle sounds such as the sound of the sea, rain or instrumental music to create a soundtrack to accompany your movements. You can find yoga-specific playlists on platforms such as **Spotify** or **YouTube**.

Fabrics

Use soft blankets or mats to make the environment cozy and comfortable. A light blanket can be useful to cover you during the final stage of relaxation (*Savasana*), keeping your body warm. Look for natural fabrics such as cotton or linen, which are pleasant to the touch and breathable. These fabrics can be found in stores such as **Zara Home** or **H&M Home**, which offer good quality products at affordable prices.

Plants Finally, add plants to the environment. Plants not only improve air quality but also instill a sense of tranquility and harmony. Plants such as ficus, sansevieria or pothos are easy to care for and have purifying properties. You can buy plants at any nursery or in the gardening departments of department stores such as **Leroy Merlin**.

With these arrangements, you will create a space that promotes relaxation not only of the body, but also of the mind, allowing you to fully immerse yourself in your yoga practice.

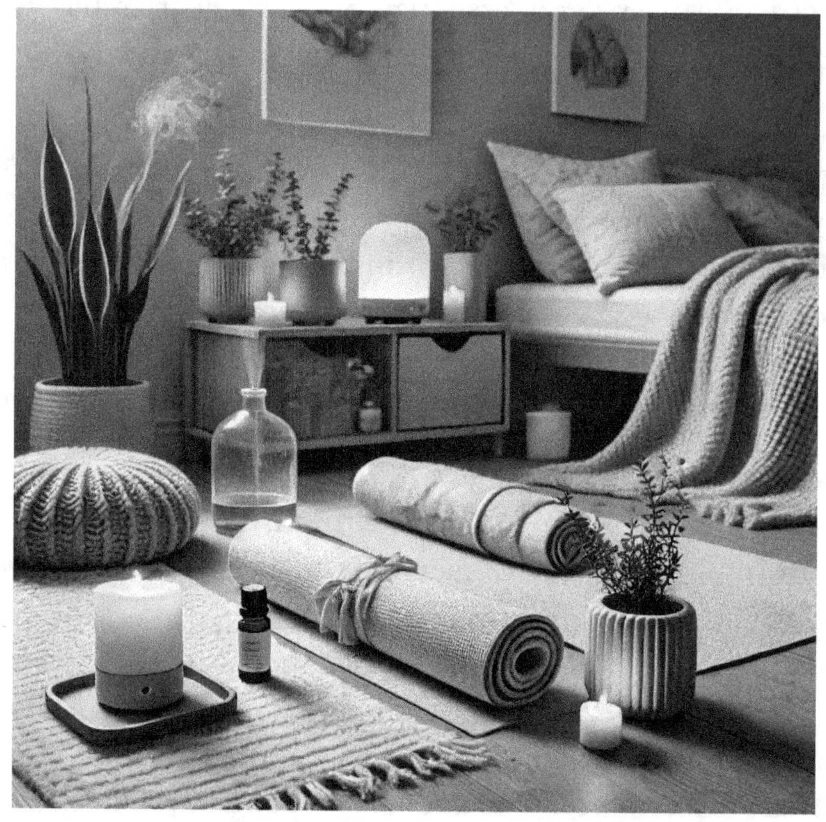

2.5 Pre-yoga practices to prepare mentally

Before you begin your yoga session, it is important to prepare yourself mentally by cultivating a state of mindfulness and calm. The way you approach your practice profoundly affects the quality of time you devote to yourself.

Mental preparation helps you get in tune with your body and mind, leaving aside daily worries.

A great place to start is to find a few minutes to sit in a comfortable position, on a pillow or directly on the mat. Close your eyes and focus on your breath. Start breathing deeply, inhaling through your nose and exhaling through your mouth. The goal is to slow the breath and make it fluid, bringing your attention inward, away from outside distractions. This initial exercise helps calm the mind, relax the body and create a deeper connection with the present moment.

During these minutes of mindful breathing, try to let go of all thoughts that are not related to your practice. Don't fight them, but imagine the thoughts flowing away like clouds in the sky. Bring your attention to the breath, the sensation of air entering and leaving the body, and how the diaphragm moves. Mentally repeat simple phrases such as, "I am present," or "I open myself to this experience," to focus your intention.

The thought you need to cultivate before the practice is one of acceptance and listening. Yoga is not about perfection, but about connecting with yourself. Cultivate in your mind the idea that you are about to take a moment just for you, without judging yourself or forcing your body beyond its limits. Practice gratitude for having the opportunity to move and breathe, even if only for a few minutes.

Another useful mental practice is to visualize the positive outcome of the session. Imagine yourself performing the postures calmly and serenely, experiencing feelings of lightness and openness. This type of visualization helps you create a positive state of mind, ready to welcome all the benefits of the practice.

Mental preparation for yoga does not take much time, but it is important to spend at least **5-10 minutes** before you begin your practice. This time is enough to calm the mind, enter a state of awareness and create the right intention for your session. <u>If you have more time, you can extend the preparation phase to **15 minutes**, especially if you feel your mind is particularly crowded or if you need to relax more deeply</u>. The important thing is that this time is devoted only to yourself, without rushing, to encourage a more focused and mindful practice.

Chapter 3: Introduction to the Weekly Yoga Program for Beginners

Goal: To create a weekly routine to introduce the practice of yoga.

3.1 Structuring a basic session: duration and objectives

When beginning to practice yoga, it is essential to create a basic session that is balanced and accessible, especially for those new to the discipline. A basic session aims to introduce the body and mind to the practice, improve flexibility, strength and awareness, without overloading the body. The ideal duration for a basic yoga session for beginners is about **20 to 30 minutes**. This time is sufficient to warm up the muscles, practice the main postures and conclude with relaxation.

Explanation of time allocation

- **First 5-7 minutes:** Warm-up and breathing. Begin each session with deep breathing exercises (*Pranayama*) and simple movements to awaken the body, such as light twists and stretches. This will help you prepare muscles and joints for later positions, while also improving concentration.

- **Middle 10-15 minutes:** Main postures. After warming up, you can focus on the main postures

(*Asana*), with a combination of exercises that involve the whole body. For beginners, it is helpful to focus on movements that improve balance, flexibility, and core strength. Postures such as the Mountain (*Tadasana*), Forward Bend (*Uttanasana*), and Warrior I (*Virabhadrasana I*) are simple but effective. The chair will be your support in these beginning stages, helping you find stability and confidence as you perform the postures.

- **Last 5-8 minutes:** Relaxation and meditation. Each session should end with a moment of deep relaxation. At this stage, postures such as Child's Posture (*Balasana*) or simply lying on the floor in *Savasana* (Corpse Posture) allow you to completely relax the body. You can also incorporate a few minutes of guided meditation or mindful breathing to calm the mind and foster the body-mind connection.

Objectives of the basic session

The basic session has some clear and simple objectives:

1. **Develop body awareness**: Learning to feel and listen to the body is fundamental in yoga. During each movement, pay attention to how your muscles move and how your body responds to each pose.

2. **Improve flexibility and strength**: Although the basic postures may seem simple, they help you work on strength and flexibility. Each session gradually and safely strengthens the body, encouraging progressive growth.

3. **Cultivating a calm and focused mind**: Yoga is not just physical movement. Working on breathing and ending the practice with a mental relaxation phase helps you maintain a clear mind, reducing stress and improving concentration.

4. **Create a sustainable routine**: The basic session should be simple enough to be repeated several times during the week. The key is consistency: even if you practice for 20 to 30 minutes a day, you will begin to notice the physical and mental benefits within the first few weeks.

A basic session structured in this way allows the beginner to begin confidently and calmly, laying the foundation for gradual and sustainable progress in yoga.

3.2 Day 1-3:

light breathing and stretching exercises

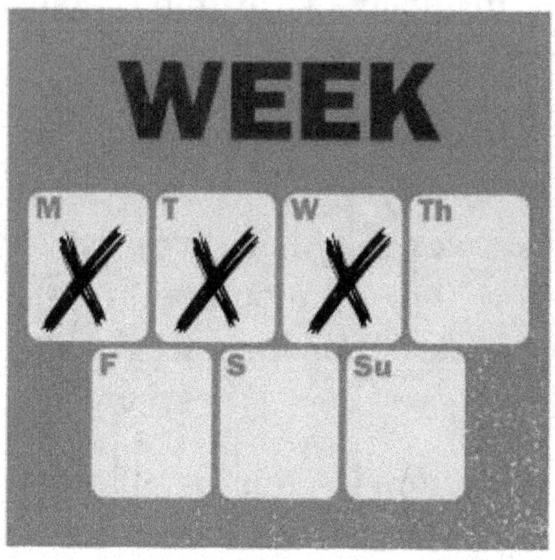

The first few days of your weekly practice are devoted to gentle breathing and stretching exercises, which are essential to awaken the body and prepare it for the more dynamic phases. The goal is to develop a deep awareness of the breath and gently stretch the muscles, improving mobility without forcing. Follow these simple exercises, step by step.

- **Exercise 1: Deep Breathing**

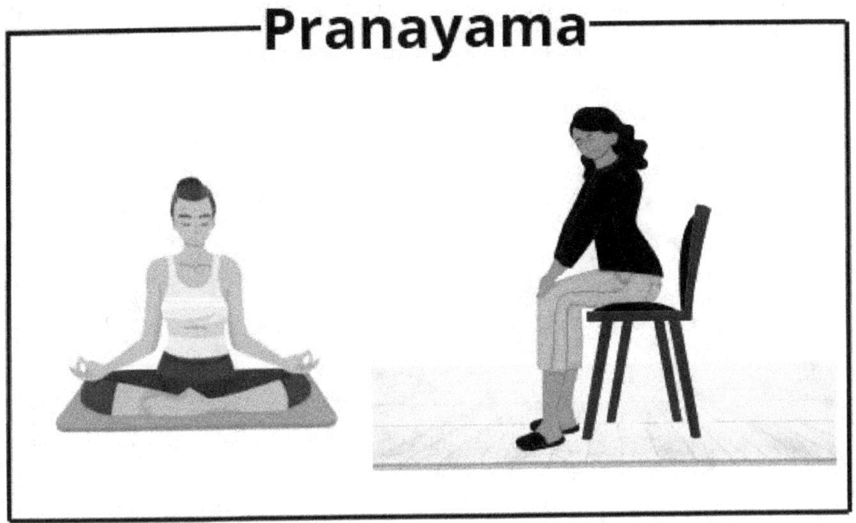

Position: Sit in a comfortable cross-legged position on the mat (as in the picture). If you prefer, you can use a chair, sitting with your feet firmly planted on the floor and your back straight.

1. Rest your hands on your knees, palms facing upward in an opening gesture. Close your eyes and relax your shoulders.

2. Begin by breathing slowly and deeply through your nose. Mentally count to 4 as you inhale, feeling the air fill your lungs and swell your abdomen.

3. Hold your breath for a couple of seconds, then exhale slowly and completely through your nose, counting to 6.

4. Repeat this deep breathing for 5-10 cycles, focusing on the sensation of air entering and leaving your body. Visualize each breath as a wave that calms the mind and body.

- **Exercise 2: Lateral stretching**

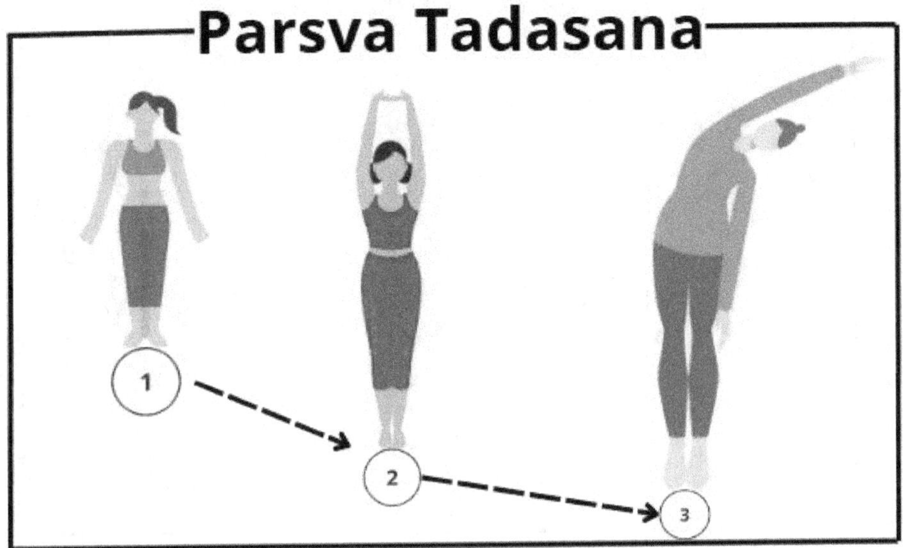

Position: Stand with feet hip-width apart.

1. Raise both arms above the head with hands touching.

2. Inhaling, stretch your body upward, as if you want to touch the ceiling.

3. As you exhale, gently tilt your torso to the right, feeling the stretch along the left side of your body. Keep the chest open and do not force.

4. Return to the center as you inhale and repeat on the left side.

5. Repeat for 4-5 cycles on each side, always keeping the breath fluid

- **Exercise 3: Stretching forward**

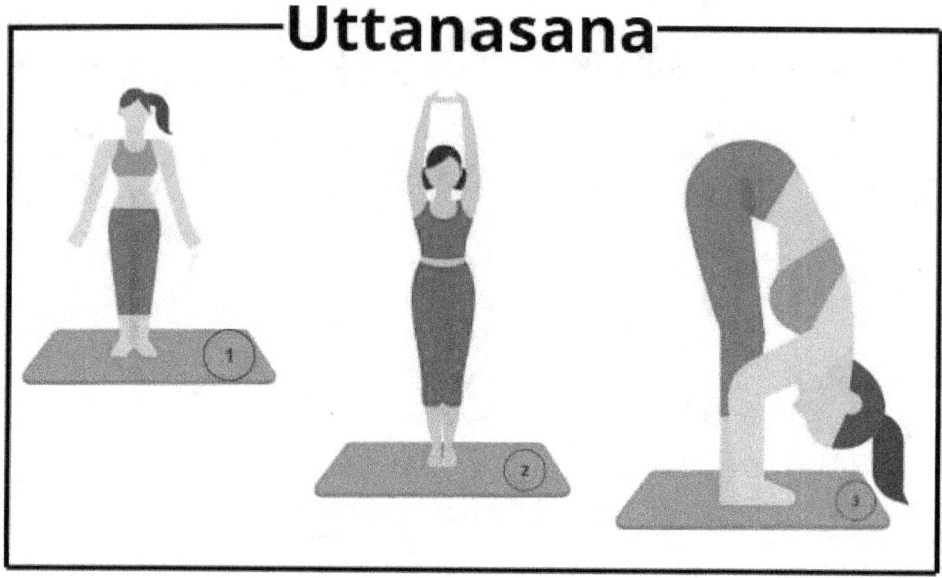

Position: Start standing, with feet slightly apart.

1. Inhaling, stretch your arms upward.

2. Exhaling, bend your torso forward from your hips, keeping your back straight as far as your body will allow. Let your hands drop to the floor, legs slightly bent if necessary.

3. It relaxes the neck and shoulders, allowing gravity to help you release tension.

4. Hold the position for 5 deep breaths, feeling the stretch in your legs and back. To exit the position, inhale and slowly return to standing, unwinding the spine.

- **Exercise 4: Seated twisting**

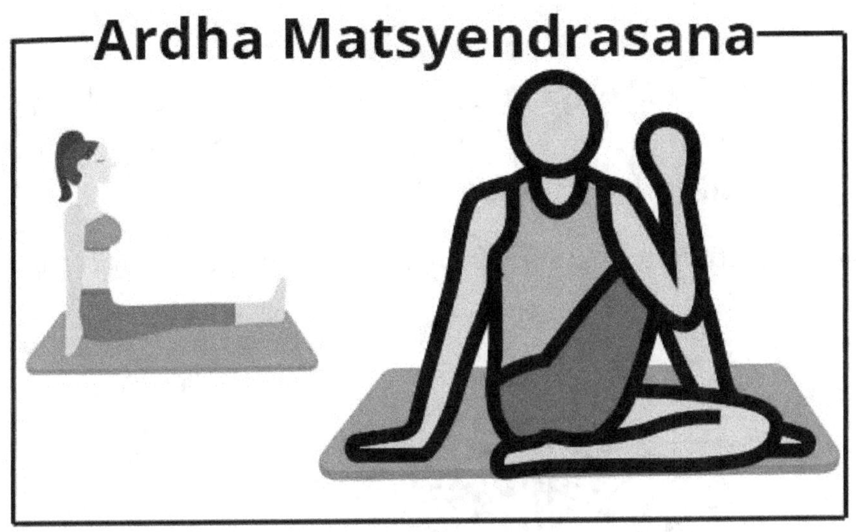

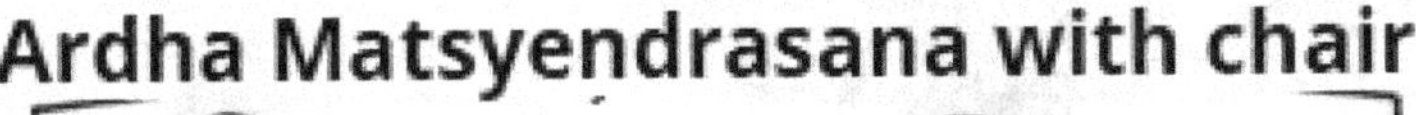

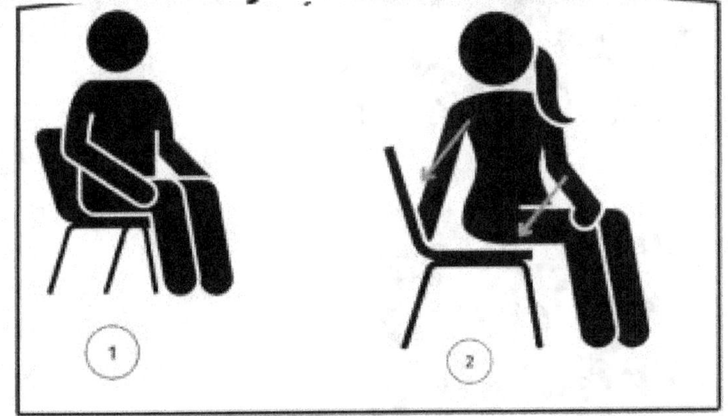

Position: Sit in a chair or on the floor with your legs crossed.

1. Inhaling, lengthen the spine upward.

2. Exhaling, slowly rotate your torso to the right, resting your left hand on your right knee (raising, if you can,

33

your right knee and bringing it to the outside of your left leg) and your right hand behind you on the chair or floor.

3. Hold the twist for 5 deep breaths, trying to lengthen the torso with each inhalation and rotate slightly more with each exhalation.

4. Return to the center by inhaling and repeat on the left side.

on the mat

on the chair

These light breathing and stretching exercises on the first three days of the program are designed to gently awaken the body and establish a connection between mind, body and breath. Regular practice of these exercises creates a solid foundation for the more challenging days that follow.

3.3 Day 4-5:

introduction to the first basic positions with the chair

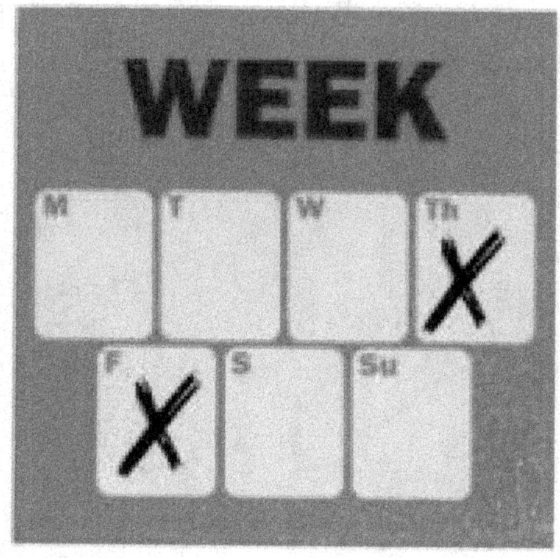

On days 4 and 5 of your program, we begin to introduce the first yoga postures using a chair. The chair will help you find stability and perform the postures safely and comfortably, especially if you are just starting out or want extra support. The postures I will explain are simple and ideal for improving balance, flexibility, and strength. Follow each step carefully and remember to breathe deeply during the exercises.

- **Position 1: Tadasana on the Chair**

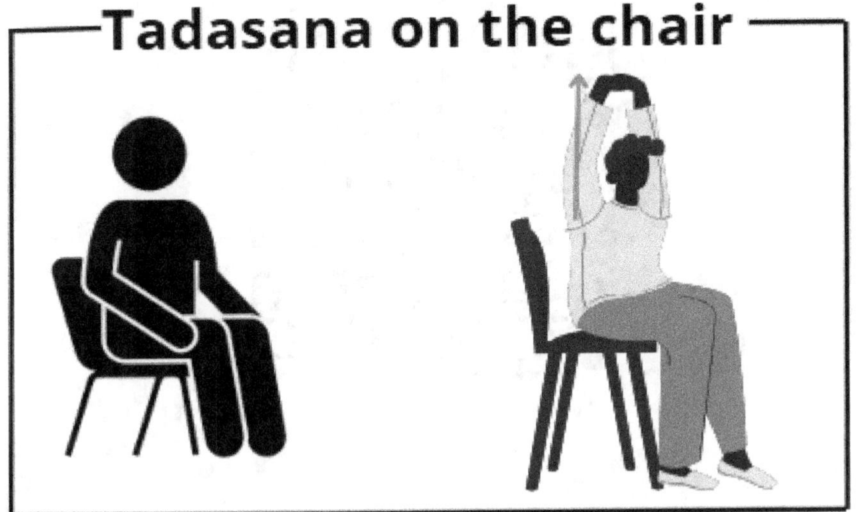

1. Sit in a chair

- Place your feet firmly on the floor, hip-width apart.

- The back is straight and the shoulders are relaxed. The hands are resting on the knees.

2. Raise the arms upward

- Inhale deeply and slowly raise your arms above your head. Your arms should be extended, but without stiffness.

- Stretch your whole body upward, as if you wanted to touch the ceiling with your fingers.

3. Hold the position

- Stay in this position for 3-5 deep breaths. Imagine yourself becoming as tall and strong as a mountain.

- Exhale and lower your arms slowly to your sides.

- **Position 2: Uttanasana Modified with chair**

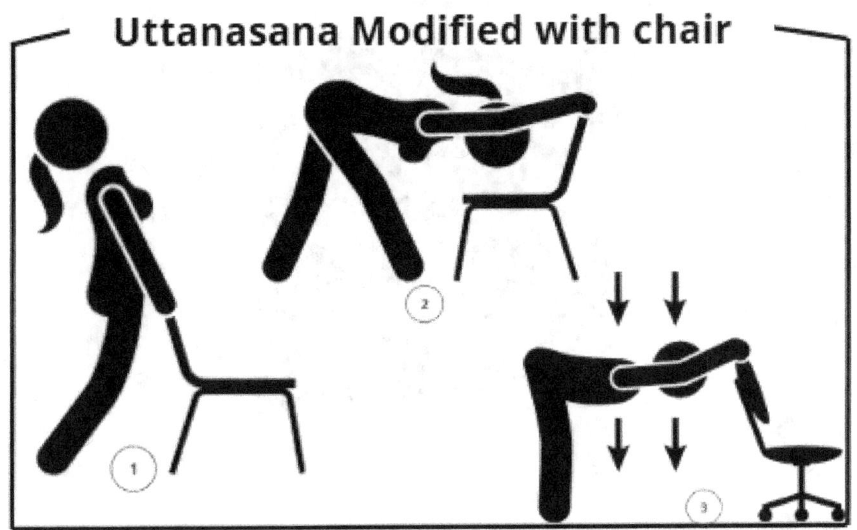

1. Stand behind the chair

- Place your hands on the back of the chair and move your feet about one step away.

2. Lean forward

- Inhaling, stretch your back. Exhaling, bend forward from the hips, keeping your back straight and resting your hands on the back of the chair for support.

- Try to bring the torso parallel to the floor.

3. Hold the position

- Hold the position for 3-5 deep breaths. You will feel a slight stretch in your back and legs.

- To exit the position, inhale and slowly return to standing.

- **Position 3: Vrksasana Modified with Chair**

Vrksasana with chair

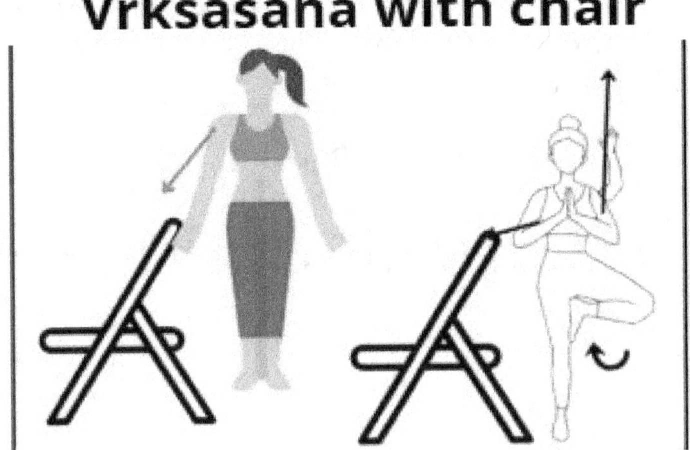

1. Stand next to the chair

- Put your right hand on the back of the chair to find balance.

2. Lift the left foot

- Gently rest your left foot on the inside of your right leg, lower if you feel unstable (can be on the ankle or calf, never on the knee).

3. Extend the left arm upward

- As you inhale, lift your left arm upward, stretching the side of your body. Try to keep your balance by helping yourself with the chair.

4. Hold the position

- Stay in position for 3-5 deep breaths, trying to feel strong and rooted like a tree. Then, repeat on the other side.

- **Position 4: Sitting in Torsion**

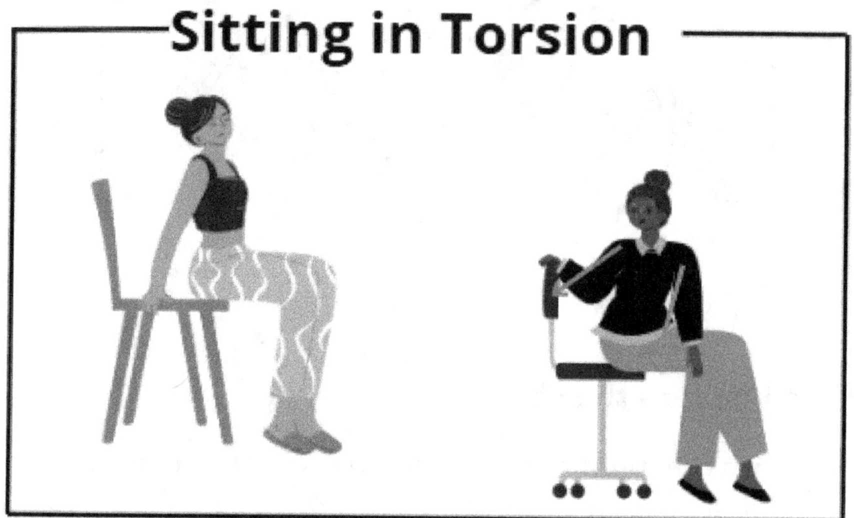

1. Sit on the edge of the chair

- Keep your feet firmly planted on the ground and your back straight.

2. Rotate the torso

- Rest your right hand on the outer side of your left knee. Place your left hand on the back of the chair.

- Inhaling, lengthen the column upward. Exhaling, gently rotate the torso to the left.

3. Hold the position

- Stay in the twist for 3-5 deep breaths. Then, return to the center and repeat on the other side.

These chair positions help you strengthen the body and improve flexibility without putting too much stress on the joints. Keep your breathing deep and steady, and remember that it doesn't matter how far you can stretch-what matters is awareness and connection with the body.

3.4 Day 6:
Full 30-minute session with focus on relaxation and breathing

On this day, we will focus on a full yoga session that lasts about 30 minutes. The main goal is to relax your body and mind, using deep breathing to feel calm and peaceful. You'll follow a simple sequence that is perfect for relaxing your muscles and banishing stress.

1. Beginning: Deep breathing (5 minutes)

Position: Sit comfortably in a chair or on a mat, with your back straight and your hands on your knees.

- Close your eyes and start breathing deeply. Inhale through your nose, counting to 4, then exhale slowly, still through your nose, counting to 6.

- Imagine that each breath relaxes you more and more. With each exhalation, let go of any tension.

- Continue for 5 minutes, keeping the focus only on the breath. If you become distracted, gently bring your attention back to the rhythm of the breath.

2. Tadasana in the chair (see previous photo) 3 minutes

Position: Sit up straight in a chair with your feet firmly planted on the floor.

- Raise your arms slowly upward, stretching your whole body as if you wanted to touch the ceiling.

- Inhale as you stretch your arms and back. Exhale as you gently lower your shoulders. Imagine you are a tall, strong mountain.

- Hold this position for 5 deep breaths. Slowly relax your arms downward.

3. Modified Uttanasana (see previous photo) 5 minutes

Position: Stand behind a chair with your hands resting on the backrest.

- Inhaling, stretch your back upward. Exhaling, slowly bend forward from the hips, keeping your back straight and knees slightly bent.

- Hold the position for 5 deep breaths, feeling the stretch in your back and legs. Return to standing position by inhaling.

5. Modified Vrksasana (see previous photo) 5 minutes

Position: Stand beside the chair, with your right hand resting on the backrest for balance.

- Lift your left foot and rest it on the inside of your right ankle or calf. Keeping your balance, raise your left arm upward.

- Hold this position for 5 deep breaths. Repeat on the other side, changing hands and feet.

6. Seated twist (see previous photo) 5 minutes

Position: Sit on the edge of the chair with your feet firmly planted on the floor.

- Rest your right hand on your left knee. Inhaling, lengthen the spine. Exhaling, slowly rotate the torso to the left.

- Hold the twist for 5 deep breaths, then return to center. Repeat on the other side.

7. Savasana on chair (Final relaxation, 7 minutes)

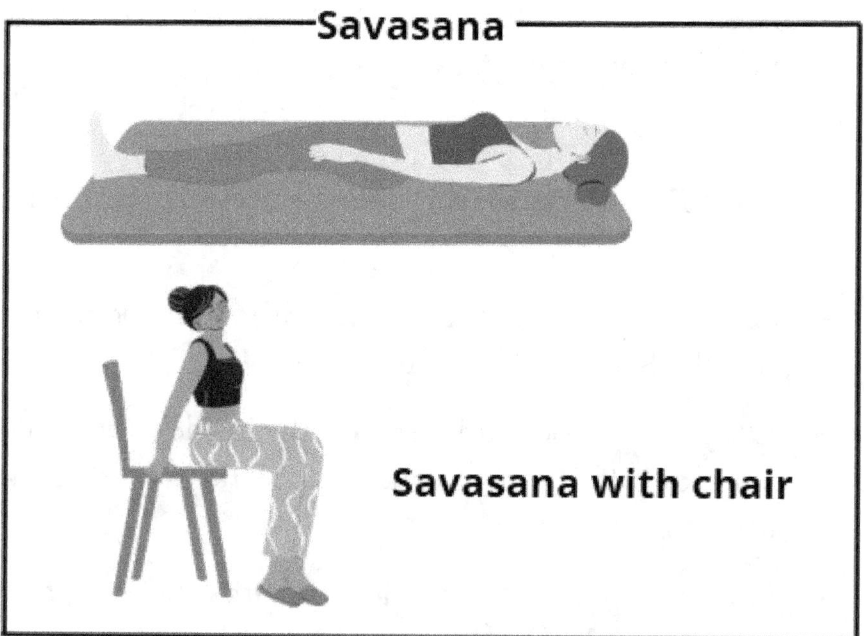

Position: Sit comfortably in a chair or lie on a mat, with your back supported and legs extended.

- Close your eyes and relax your body completely.
  Imagine the entire weight of your body melting into
  the chair or the floor.

- Breathe slowly and deeply. Each time you exhale,
  imagine letting go of any tension or thoughts.

- Stay in this position of complete relaxation for 7
  minutes, focusing only on your breath and the sense
  of peace that pervades you.

After 30 minutes of practice, you should feel calm, relaxed
and more in touch with your body. This sequence helps you
not only to relax physically, but also to calm your mind,
allowing you to face the day or evening with serenity and
clarity. Remember that yoga is not about how far you can
stretch, but rather about the awareness and calmness you
cultivate during practice.

<u>**3.5 Day 7:**</u>

<u>**rest and reflection on the week of practice**</u>

Today is your day of rest! You will not do physical exercises, but we will focus on relaxation and reflection. This is an important time to allow your body to recover and your mind to take a break. Even if you don't practice yoga postures today, you can still take a few minutes to think about how the week went and how you felt after each practice. By following these steps, I will guide you through a time of reflection and relaxation.

1. Find a quiet place to reflect (5 minutes)

- Sit in a place where you feel comfortable and relaxed. You can sit in a chair, on a mat, or even on a bed.

- Close your eyes and take a few deep breaths, just as you learned in previous days.

- Inhale slowly through your nose, feel your chest expand, then exhale slowly through your mouth. Do this five times.

2. Reflection on the week's practice (10 minutes)

Now is the time to think about your week of yoga. I will ask you some questions and you can answer them for yourself, reflecting on how you felt.

- **How did you feel after the first day of breathing and stretching?**

- Did you notice any changes in your body? Did you feel more calm or relaxed? Which body parts did you feel most active?

- **How did you feel when you used the chair for the basic positions?**
- Did you find the chair useful? Did you feel more confident in performing the positions? What was your favorite position?
- **Have you noticed any difference in your mind or body?**
- Do you feel more relaxed than at the beginning of the week? What have you noticed in the way you breathe, move or think during the day?

This reflection helps you become aware of the small progress you have made, even if it seems insignificant. Each day of practice brings improvement, both physical and mental, and thinking about it helps you become more self-aware.

3. Guided relaxation (10 minutes)

Now, I will guide you through a short relaxation for the body and mind.

- Sit or lie down in a comfortable position. If you are sitting, rest your back and relax your arms on your legs or hips. If you are lying down, fully stretch your arms and legs.

- Close your eyes and start breathing deeply. With each exhalation, imagine letting go of all tension.

- Now focus on your toes. Relax them. Then move on to your feet, legs and so on, moving up to your head. Imagine every part of your body becoming light and relaxed.

- When you get to your head, relax your forehead and let the thoughts flow away, like clouds in the sky. There is no need to do anything, just breathe and relax.

4. Gratitude (5 minutes)

When you have finished the relaxation, take a moment to think about something you are grateful for.

- It can be something small, like the fact that you had time to do yoga this week, or something big, like the support of the people around you.

- Being grateful for what we have makes us feel happier and more at peace with ourselves.

This rest day is the perfect time to appreciate your commitment and mentally prepare yourself for the next week of practice. Rest is also an important part of yoga!

Chapter 4: Progressions and Increasing Difficulty

4.1 Day 1:

Introduction to positions
of warm-up and stretching

Today we begin a new week of practice, and we will start with exercises that warm up the body and stretch the muscles. Warming up is very important because it prepares the body for more challenging exercises, helping you to avoid injury and improve your flexibility. I will guide you step by step through some simple positions that will make you feel ready to continue with the practice.

- **1. Deep breathing and preparation (3 minutes)**

Position: Sit comfortably, in a chair or on a mat, with your back straight.

- Close your eyes and put your hands on your knees. Breathe deeply. Breathe in slowly through your nose and feel your belly swell.

- Exhale slowly, imagining all the stress leaving your body.

- Repeat this for 5 breaths, trying to relax the shoulders and neck.

- **2. Arm extension, 3 minutes**

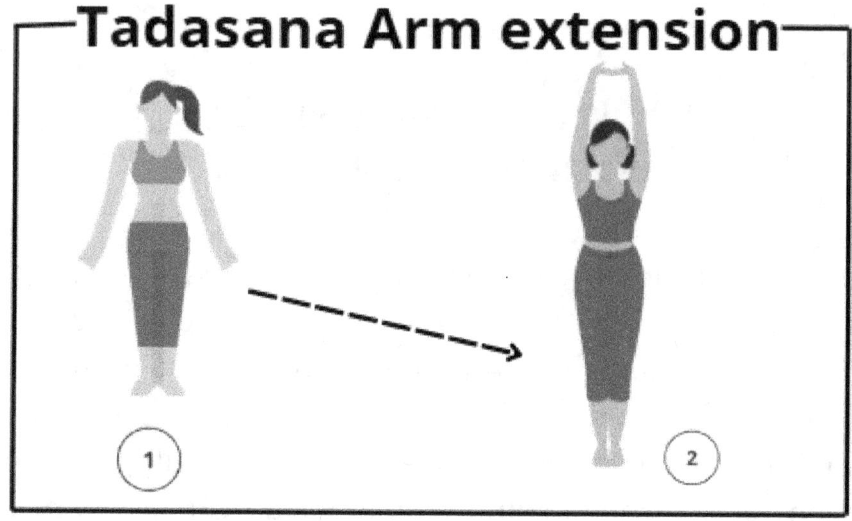

Position: Standing with feet hip-width apart.

- Inhaling, slowly lift your arms upward, stretching your fingers toward the ceiling. Stretch as if you want to become taller.

- Hold the position for 5 deep breaths, feeling your whole body stretch, from your toes to your hands.

- Exhaling, slowly lower the arms. Repeat for 3 times.

- **3. Side bending, 4 minutes**

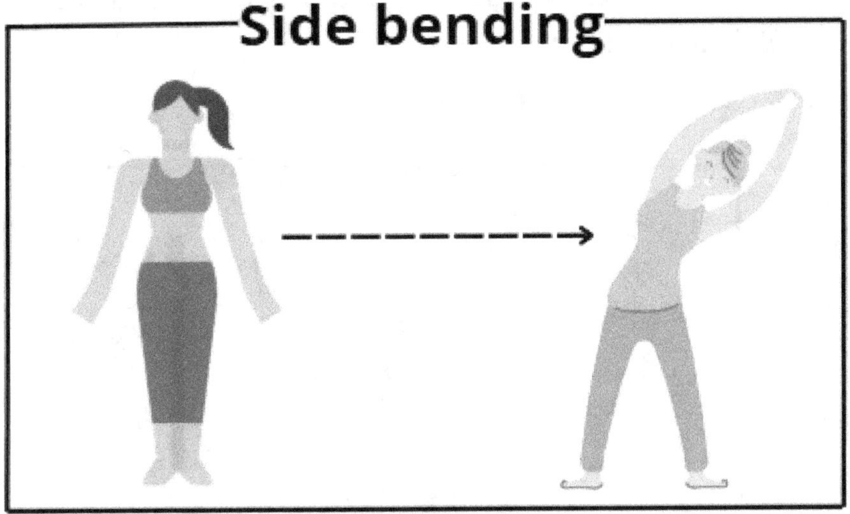

Position: Stand with your feet shoulder-width apart and your arms along your sides.

- Inhaling, raise the right arm upward. Exhaling, slowly bend the torso to the left, feeling the stretch along the right side of the body.

- Hold the position for 3 breaths, then return to center by inhaling.

- Repeat on the other side, with the left arm overhead. Do this 3 times on each side.

- **4. Forward bending (Uttanasana), 5 minutes, Without chair**

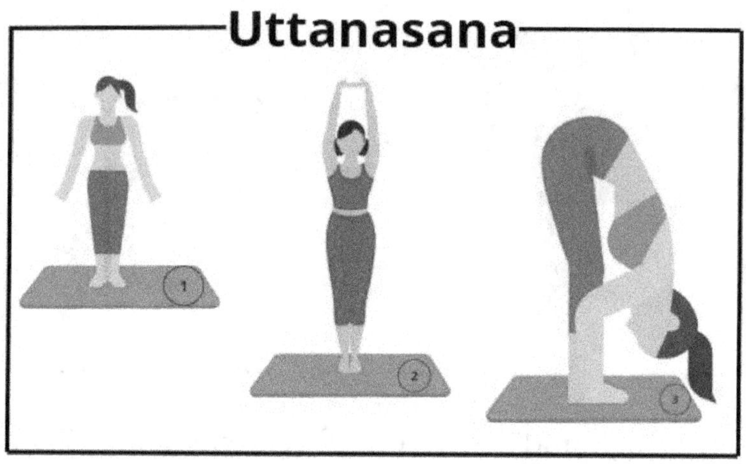

Position: Standing, with feet slightly apart.

- Inhaling, lift your arms upward. Exhaling, bend forward from the hips, letting the arms descend toward the floor.

- If you cannot touch the floor, it is perfectly fine to bend your knees. The important thing is that your neck and back are relaxed.

- Hold the position for 5 deep breaths. Then, inhaling, return to standing slowly.

- **5. Gentle twist (Seated twist) 5 minutes**

SEE PREVIOUS IMAGE

Position: Sit in a chair with your feet firmly planted on the floor.

- Inhaling, stretch your back. Exhaling, gently rotate your torso to the right, resting your left hand on your right knee and your right hand on the back of the chair.

- Hold position for 5 deep breaths, then return to center. Repeat on the opposite side.

These exercises are perfect for warming up your muscles and stretching your body. Don't rush: the key is to breathe deeply and enjoy each movement. With these simple steps, your body will be ready for more advanced positions!

4.2 Day 2:
Focus on the core with light exercises using the chair

Today we are going to focus on the *core*, that is, the belly and back muscles. These muscles are very important because they help you keep your balance and stand up straight. For these exercises, we will use a chair to give you stability and support. Don't worry if you find them a little difficult at first-the key is to practice calmly and with concentration.

- **1.Lifting knees while sitting (5 minutes)**

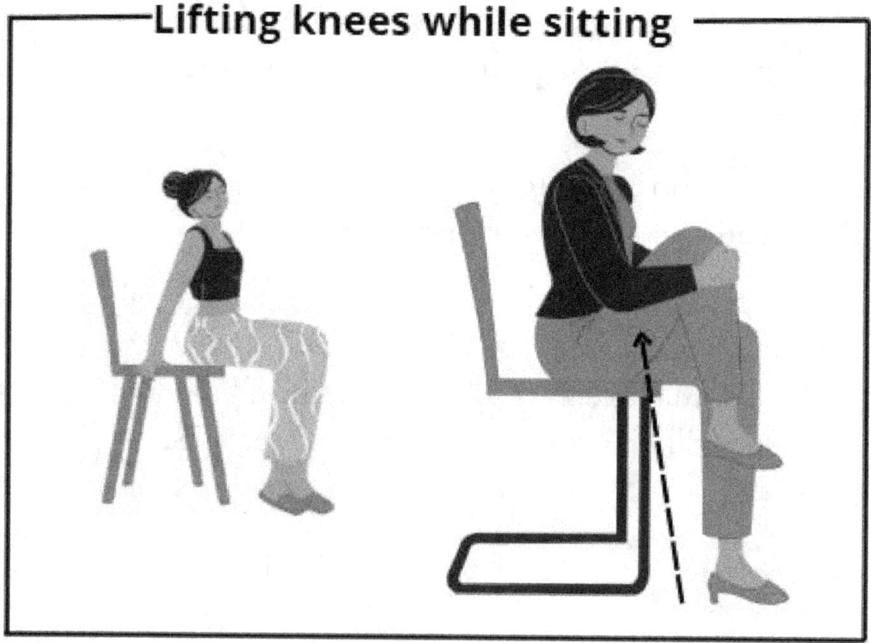

Position: Sit in a chair with your back straight, feet firmly on the floor and hands on your hips or knees.

- Inhale deeply. Exhaling, slowly lift your right knee toward your chest, keeping your left foot firmly planted on the ground.

- Keep your back straight and try not to move too much. Hold your knee up for 3 deep breaths, then slowly lower it.

- Repeat the same movement with the left leg. Alternate legs 5 times on each side.

- **2.Modified plank with chair (5 minutes)**

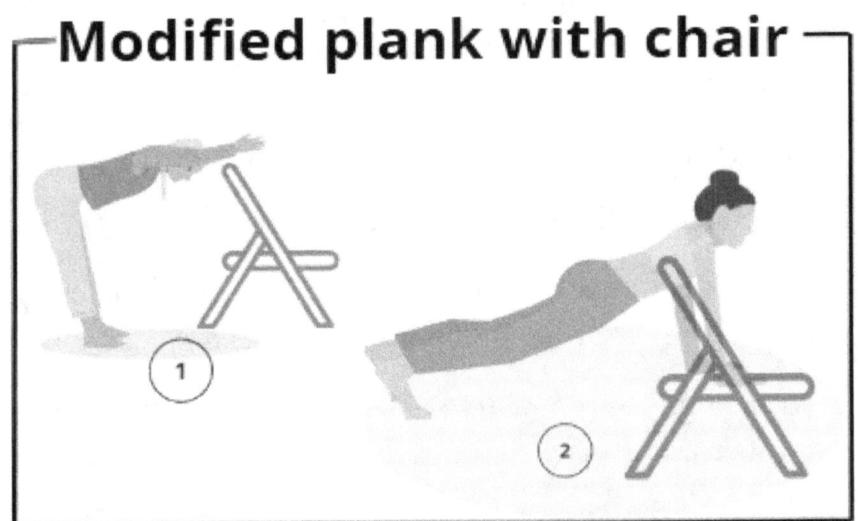

Position: Stand behind the chair or in front, with your hands resting on the backrest or you can lean on the inside of the chair.

- Move your feet away from the chair so that your body is slightly tilted. Your body should form a straight line from your shoulders to your feet.

- Contract your belly muscles, keeping your body still. Breathe deeply and try not to arch your back.

- Hold the position for 3-5 deep breaths, then slowly return to the starting position. Repeat 3 times.

- **3. Seated twists for the core (5 minutes)**

  SEE PREVIOUS IMAGE

Position: Sit on the edge of the chair with your feet resting on the floor and your hands behind your head.

- Inhaling, stretch your back. Exhaling, gently rotate your torso to the right, without moving your hips or legs.

- Hold the twist for 3 deep breaths, then return to center. Repeat the same movement on the left side.

- Perform 5 twists on each side.

- **4. Leg lifts from a seated position (5 minutes)**

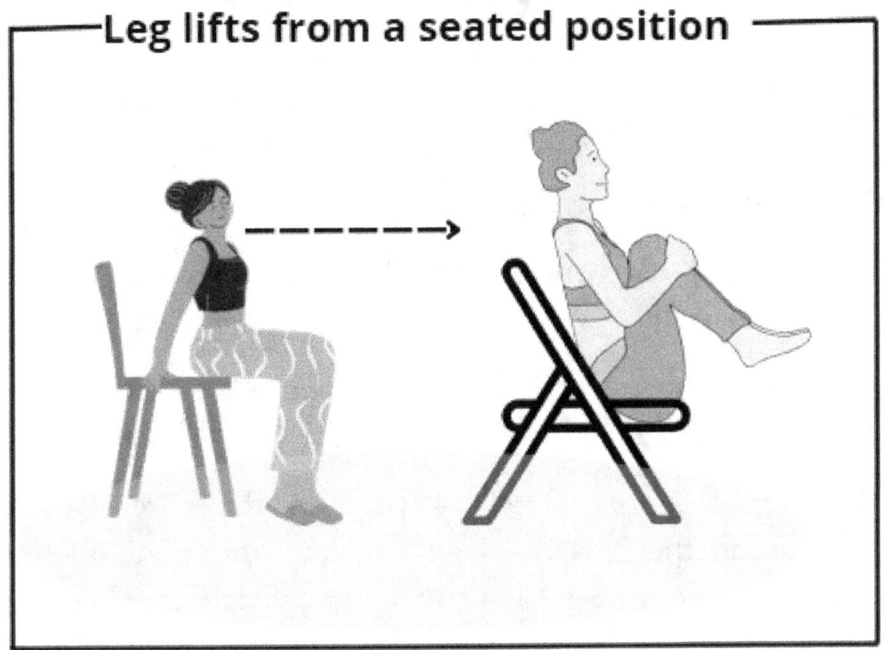

Position: Sit up straight in the chair with your hands resting on your hips.

- Inhaling, lift both legs off the ground, keeping them together and bent. Bring the knees toward the chest.

- Hold the position for 2 deep breaths, then slowly lower your legs to the floor.

- Repeat this movement 5 times. If it is too difficult, you can lift one leg at a time.

- **5. Final stretch (5 minutes)**

Position: Sit comfortably in the chair.

- Raise both arms toward the ceiling, stretching your back well.

- Hold the position for 3 deep breaths, then lower your arms and relax your whole body.

These light exercises help strengthen the core without overloading the body. Take your time and remember to breathe deeply during each movement. Strengthening your core will help you improve your balance and posture!

<u>**4.3 Day 3:**</u>

<u>**Toning exercises for legs and buttocks**</u>

Today we are going to focus on the *core*, that is, the belly and back muscles. These muscles are very important because they help you keep your balance and stand up straight. For these exercises, we will use a chair to give you stability and support. Don't worry if you find them a little difficult at first-the key is to practice calmly and with concentration.

1. Lifting knees from a seated position

(5 minutes)

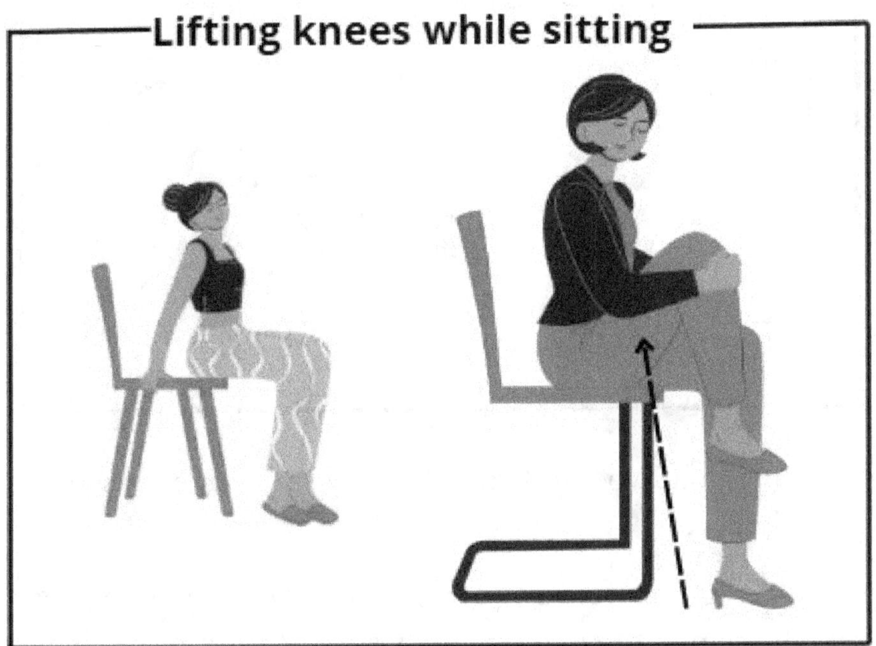

Position: Sit in a chair with your back straight, feet firmly on the floor and hands on your hips or knees.

- Inhale deeply. Exhaling, slowly lift your right knee toward your chest, keeping your left foot firmly planted on the ground.

- Keep your back straight and try not to move too much. Hold your knee up for 3 deep breaths, then slowly lower it.

- Repeat the same movement with the left leg. Alternate legs 5 times on each side.

2. Modified plank with chair (5 minutes)

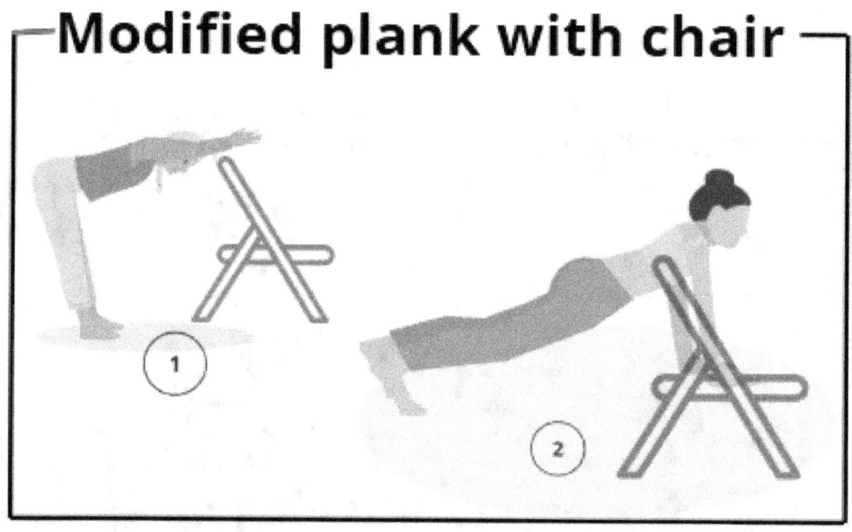

Position: Stand behind the chair, with your hands resting on the backrest.

- Move your feet away from the chair so that your body is slightly tilted. Your body should form a straight line from your shoulders to your feet.

- Contract your belly muscles, keeping your body still. Breathe deeply and try not to arch your back.

- Hold the position for 3-5 deep breaths, then slowly return to the starting position. Repeat 3 times.

3. Sitting twists for the core (5 minutes)

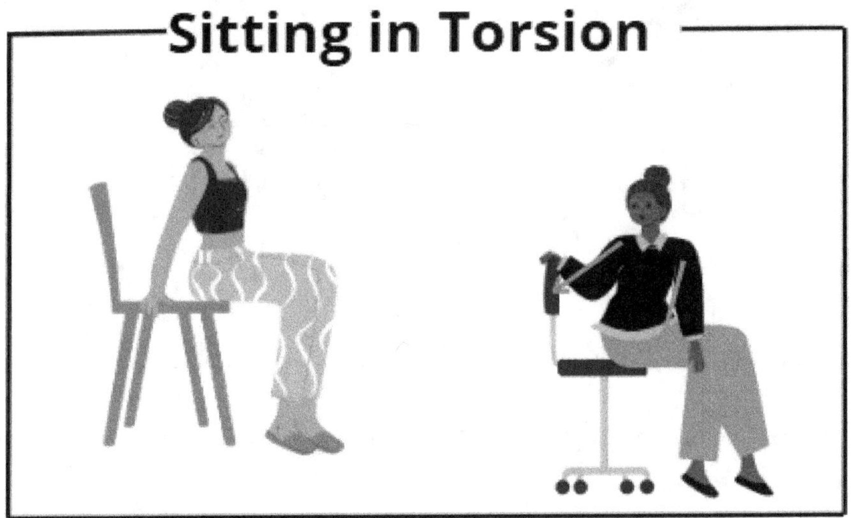

Position: Sit on the edge of the chair with your feet resting on the floor and your hands behind your head.

- Inhaling, stretch your back. Exhaling, gently rotate your torso to the right, without moving your hips or legs.

- Hold the twist for 3 deep breaths, then return to center. Repeat the same movement on the left side.

- Perform 5 twists on each side.

4. Leg lifts from a seated position (5 minutes)

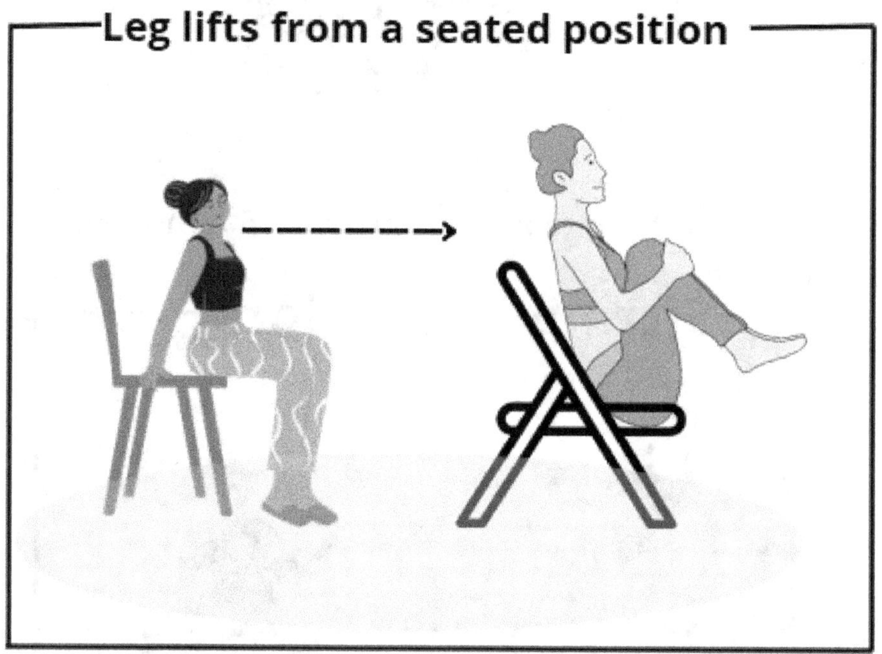

Position: Sit up straight in the chair with your hands resting on your hips.

- Inhaling, lift both legs off the ground, keeping them together and bent. Bring the knees toward the chest.

- Hold the position for 2 deep breaths, then slowly lower your legs to the floor.

- Repeat this movement 5 times. If it is too difficult, you can lift one leg at a time.

5. Final stretch (5 minutes)

Position: Sit comfortably in the chair.

- Raise both arms toward the ceiling, stretching your back well.

- Hold the position for 3 deep breaths, then lower your arms and relax your whole body.

These light exercises help strengthen the core without overloading the body. Take your time and remember to breathe deeply during each movement. Strengthening your core will help you improve your balance and posture!

<u>4.4 Day 4:</u>

<u>Toning exercises for arms and shoulders</u>

Today we will focus on arms and shoulders. These muscles help you lift objects, maintain good posture and move with ease. We will use a chair to give support and safety during the exercises. Follow along step by step, and remember to do the movements slowly, carefully and while breathing deeply.

1. Arm lifts (5 minutes)

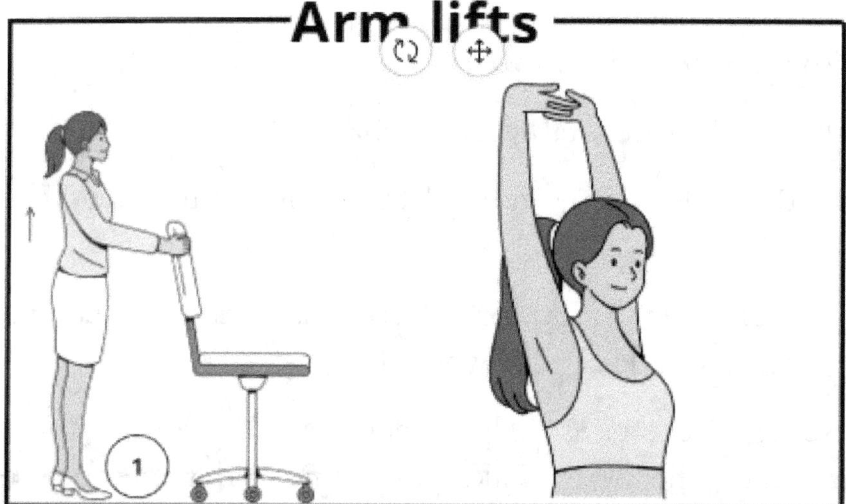

Position: Stand behind chair with feet hip-width apart.

- Gently rest your hands on the back of the chair. Inhaling, slowly lift both arms upward, as if you want to touch the ceiling.

- As you lift your arms, stretch your shoulders well and feel the stretch in your muscles.

- Exhale by lowering your arms slowly to the sides of your body. Repeat this movement 8-10 times, trying to stretch a little more each time.

2. Modified chair push-ups (5 minutes)

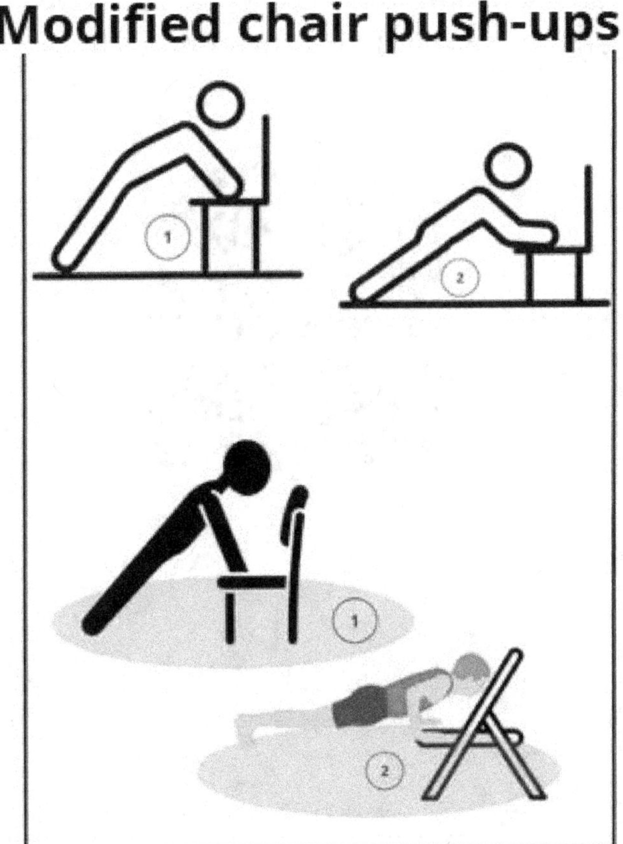

Position: Stand in front of the chair, with your hands resting on the inside of the chair.

- Move your feet away from the chair so that your body is slightly tilted. Your hands remain firmly on the seat, aligned with your shoulders.

- Inhaling, slowly bend your elbows and lower yourself toward the chair, as if you were going to do a push-up. Keep your body straight and your elbows close to your sides.

- Exhale by pushing the body back until you return to an upright position. Repeat for 6 to 8 times.

3. Shoulder circumduction (5 minutes)

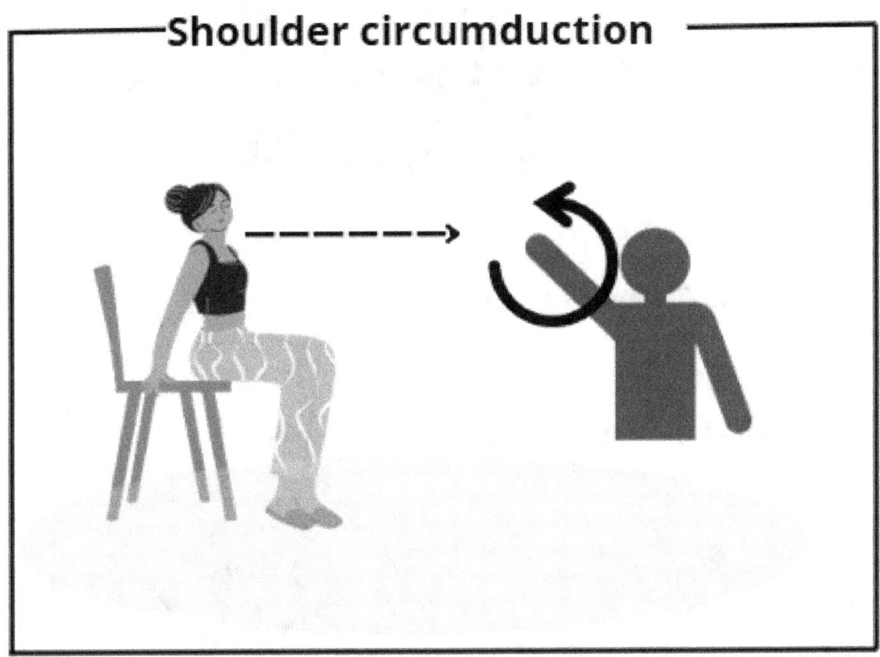

Position: Sit in the chair with your feet firmly planted on the floor.

- Rest your hands on your knees. Breathing in, make a circular motion with your shoulders, lifting them toward your ears and then moving them back, as if you were going to make circles.

- Repeat for 5 circles forward and 5 circles backward, breathing deeply and relaxing the neck.

4. Arm stretching (5 minutes)

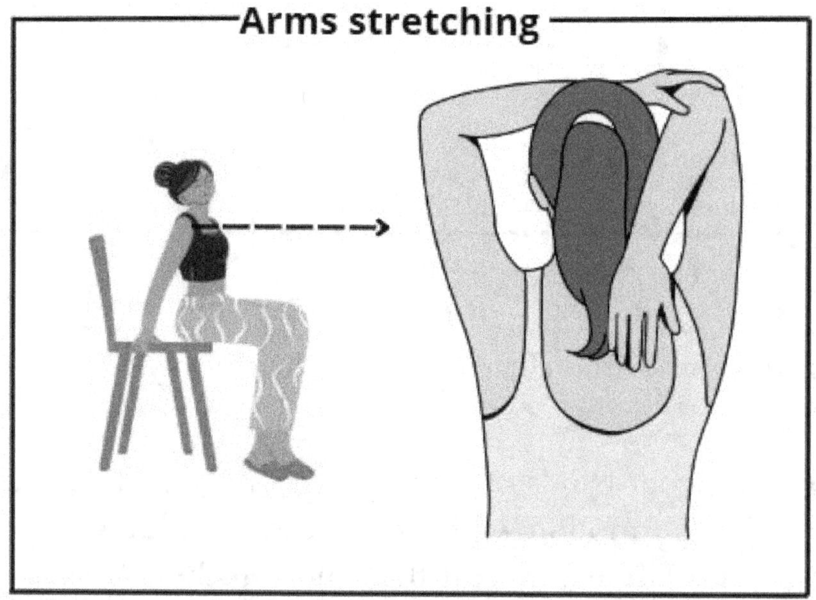

Position: Sit in the chair with your back straight.

- Raise your right arm above your head, then bend it behind your back as if to touch your left shoulder.

- With your left hand, gently take your right elbow and pull slightly, feeling the stretch in your shoulder and arm.

- Hold the position for 3 deep breaths, then repeat on the other side.

5. Final Stretch (5 minutes)

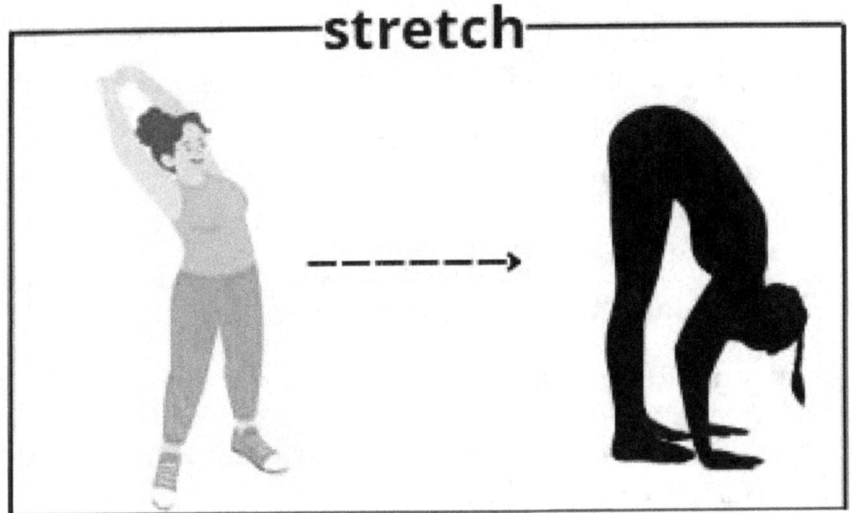

Position: Stand with feet shoulder-width apart.

- Inhaling, lift both arms upward. Exhaling, bend your torso forward, letting your arms descend toward the floor.

- Hold the position for 3 breaths, then slowly rise again. Repeat 3 times.

These simple exercises will help you strengthen your arms and shoulders, improving your strength and endurance. Don't forget to do each movement calmly and breathe deeply, so you'll help your muscles work better!

4.5 Day 5:
Complete stretching and conscious breathing

Today we are going to do some full-body stretching along with mindful breathing. Stretching helps make muscles more flexible, while mindful breathing helps us relax the mind and focus on the present. Follow step by step, and remember to always breathe calmly and deeply.

1. Deep breathing to start (3 minutes)

Position: Sit comfortably in a chair or on a mat.

- Close your eyes and place your hands on your knees. Start breathing slowly.

- Inhale deeply through your nose counting to 4, feeling the air fill your belly.

- Exhale slowly through the mouth, counting to 6, letting go of all tension.

- Do this for 5 breaths, focusing only on the breath movement.

2. Stretching arms above the head (5 minutes) see previous photo

Position: Stand with feet shoulder-width apart.

- Inhaling, slowly raise both arms toward the ceiling, stretching as far as possible.

- As you exhale, relax your arms and slowly lower them to the sides of your body.

- Repeat this movement 5 times, stretching a little more each time. Try to feel the stretch along the sides of your body and shoulders.

3. Forward bending (Uttanasana, 5 minutes) see previous photo

Position: Standing with feet slightly apart.

- Inhaling, stretch your arms upward. Exhaling, slowly bend forward from the hips, letting the arms descend toward the floor.

- Keep knees slightly bent if necessary. Let your head and arms be completely relaxed.

- Stay in this position for 5 deep breaths, feeling the stretch in your back and legs.

4. Lateral stretching (5 minutes) see previous photo

Position: Standing with feet shoulder-width apart.

- Inhaling, lift the right arm upward. Exhaling, bend the torso gently to the left, feeling the stretch along the right side of the body.

- Hold the position for 3 deep breaths, then return to the center and repeat on the other side with the left arm.

- Repeat 3 times on each side.

6. Neck stretching (5 minutes)

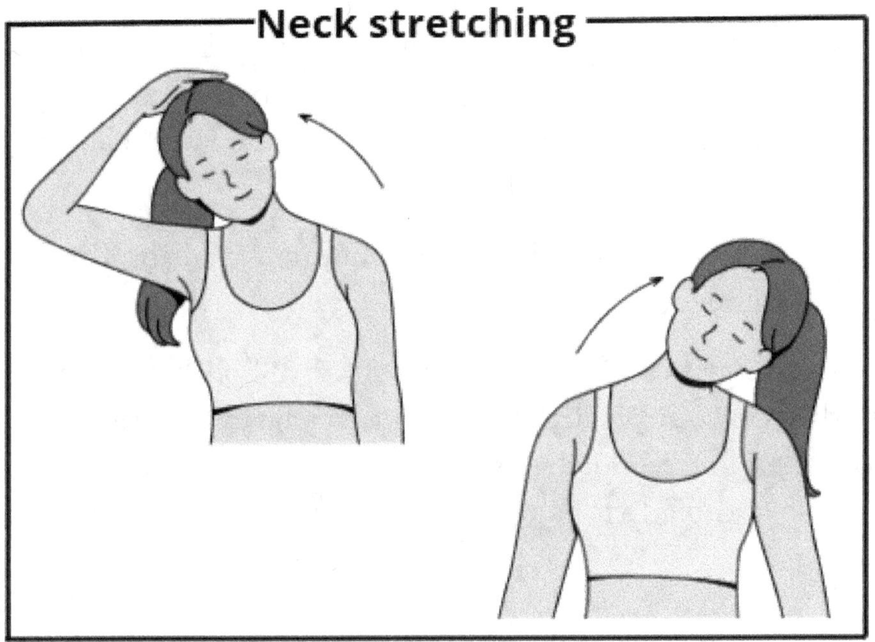

Position: Sit comfortably in a chair or on a mat.

- Tilt your head slowly to the right, trying to bring your right ear close to your right shoulder, without raising your shoulder.

- Hold the position for 3 deep breaths, then return to the center and repeat on the left side.

- After stretching your neck on both sides, make small circles with your head to further relax your neck and shoulders.

6. Conclusion with conscious breathing (5 minutes)

Position: Sit comfortably again with your hands resting on your knees.

- Close your eyes and breathe deeply. Each time you inhale, imagine that you are bringing energy and freshness into your body. Each time you exhale, let go of any tension or thoughts.

- Hold this breathing for 5 minutes, focusing only on the breath.

By this sequence, you will have done a full body stretch and worked on your breathing. Remember that each breath helps you relax more and that stretching makes your body more flexible and ready to take on more challenges!

4.6 Day 6:
Regenerative yoga sequence with final meditation

Today we are going to do a very gentle yoga sequence, called *regenerative*, which helps you relax completely and regain energy. At the end of the practice we will also do a meditation to calm the mind and find peace. These exercises are perfect for easing tension after a week of practice. Just follow the steps and breathe deeply.

1. Deep breathing and initial relaxation (3 minutes)

Position: Sit comfortably in a chair or on the mat.

- Close your eyes and place your hands on your knees. Inhale slowly through your nose, feeling the air fill your belly.

- Exhale slowly through the mouth, letting go of all tension.

- Repeat for 5 deep breaths, trying to calm the mind and prepare yourself for the practice.

2. Modified child's position (Balasana, 5 minutes)

Position: Sit in the chair, bending your upper body forward.

- Rest your head and arms on the table in front of you or on your legs. If you want, you can use a pillow to rest your head and make the position more comfortable.

- Hold the position for 5 deep breaths, feeling the body relax more and more with each exhalation.

3. Forward bending with chair (modified Uttanasana, 5 minutes)

Position: Stand behind the chair, with hands resting on the backrest.

- Inhaling, stretch your back upward. Exhaling, bend forward from the hips, letting the torso stretch parallel to the floor.

- Hold the position for 5 deep breaths, feeling the stretch in your back and legs.

- Slowly return to standing as you inhale.

4. Torsion regenerative session (5 minutes)

Position: Sit comfortably in the chair with your feet firmly planted on the floor.

- Inhaling, stretch your back. Exhaling, gently rotate your torso to the right, resting your left hand on your right knee and your right hand on the back of the chair.

- Hold the twist for 5 deep breaths, relaxing the shoulders. Then return to the center and repeat on the other side.

5. Savasana in the chair (Final relaxation, 7 minutes)

Position: Sit comfortably in the chair, leaning your back against the backrest and relaxing your arms along your sides.

- Close your eyes and let your whole body relax. Imagine the weight of your body melting into the chair.

- Breathe deeply and slowly, feeling the air gently entering and leaving. With each exhalation, relax each part of the body more and more.

- Stay in this position for 5-7 minutes, doing nothing but breathing and relaxing.

6. Final meditation (5 minutes)

- Remain in a sitting position with your eyes closed. Bring all your attention to the breath.

- Inhale counting to 4, exhale counting to 6. Imagine that you are immersed in a peaceful and serene place where nothing disturbs you.

- If thoughts come, imagine they are passing clouds and let them go. You don't have to do anything, just observe and breathe.

This restorative yoga sequence, along with meditation, will help you regain calm and energy. It is perfect for ending a busy day or a week of intense practice. Remember that relaxation is as important a part of yoga as movement!

4.7 Day 7:
Active rest day, with mindfulness tips

Today is your active rest day. This means that we will not do strenuous exercises, but will focus on moving your body in a gentle and mindful way. In addition, I will guide you through some mindfulness (awareness) techniques, which will help you be more present and relaxed. Even if it is a rest day, moving a little and practicing mindfulness can make you feel calmer and happier.

1. Mindful walking (10 minutes)

If you can, take a short walk, even if it is just indoors. This walk will be special because we will do it slowly and carefully.

- As you walk, feel your feet touching the floor. Walk slowly, trying to notice each step.
- Focus your attention on how your legs, feet and arms move. Inhale as you take a step, and exhale as you take another step.
- If you get distracted, that's okay. Gently bring your attention back to the way you are walking and breathing.

2. Gentle stretching of the back (5 minutes)

Position: Stand or sit in a chair with a straight back.

- Inhaling, stretch your arms toward the ceiling, as if you want to get taller. Feel the stretch in your back and shoulders.
- Exhaling, relax your arms at the sides of your body. Repeat 5-6 times, breathing slowly and focusing on each movement.

3. Conscious listening exercise (5 minutes)

Now we are going to do a little exercise for the mind. This will help you calm your thoughts and focus on the present.

- Sit comfortably, close your eyes and breathe deeply.

- Start listening to the sounds around you. No matter what sounds you hear, the important thing is to focus on them. You can hear wind, people, or maybe just silence.
- Don't judge the sounds. Simply listen and let them come and go.

4. Gratitude (5 minutes)

Practicing gratitude means thinking about something positive you have in your life. This helps you feel happier and more at peace.

- Close your eyes and think of three things you are grateful for. They can be small, like the food you ate today, or big, like a special person in your life.
- Breathing deeply, feel this gratitude growing inside you. Keep a smile as you think about these things, letting them fill you with joy.

5. Conclusion

This active rest day is dedicated to the well-being of your body and mind. Even if you have not done strenuous exercises, you have learned to move and be more aware of the present. *Mindfulness* helps you live each moment more calmly and gratefully, and this makes your days more beautiful and relaxed.

Chapter 5: Creating the Monthly Yoga for Weight Loss Program

5.1 How to vary the weekly schedule in the first two weeks

In the first two weeks of your monthly yoga for weight loss program, the goal is to become familiar with the postures and begin to feel stronger and more flexible. I will guide you through the modifications and variations you can make to the weekly program you have already been following, adding new challenges without overdoing it. Remember that every small step counts, and the important thing is to be consistent.

Week 1: Consolidating the basics

The first week of the monthly program is devoted to consolidating what you have learned. We won't make any big changes, but we will add a few small elements to make the practice smoother and slightly more challenging.

Days 1-3: Breathing and Stretching

Continue to focus on breathing and stretching exercises as you did in your weekly routine, but this time try to hold the stretching positions a little longer.

- **Side Extension Position**: Hold the stretch for 5-6 deep breaths, trying to stretch the side of the body even more each time you inhale.

- **Uttanasana (bending forward)**: When you bend forward, try bending your knees a little less than before, feeling a slight stretch in your leg muscles.

Day 4-5: Core exercises

Now that you are familiar with core exercises, you can add a little challenge by increasing the number of repetitions.

- **Seated Knee** Lift: Try lifting both legs together instead of one at a time, keeping your breathing fluid. Do this for 8-10 repetitions.

- **Modified plank with chair**: Hold the position for 5-7 deep breaths, contract the belly muscles well and try to keep the body aligned.

Day 6: Relaxation session with deeper stretching

Repeat the regenerative sequence you learned, but this time try to spend more time on the final relaxation (*Savasana*). Sit or lie down for at least 10 minutes, focusing only on the breath and relaxation of each part of the body.

Day 7: Rest and reflection

Keep the day active by reflecting on the small progress you have made. Remember that change takes time and perseverance.

- **<u>Week 2: Adding intensity and new challenges</u>**

In the second week, we start to make the program a little more dynamic and challenging, but always in a gradual way. We add some variations to the positions and increase the duration of some sequences.

Day 1-3: Deeper stretching positions

These days, we will focus on stretches, but we will try to make the positions slightly deeper.

- **Tadasana with arms raised**: After raising your arms above your head, try bending sideways more intensely. Keep your torso extended and take 7 deep breaths on each side.

- **Forward bend (Uttanasana)**: If you feel comfortable, try keeping your legs straighter and touching the floor with your hands without bending your knees too much. Don't force, but listen to your body.

Day 4-5: Intensify core work

For the core, we will make the exercises a little more intense this week:

- **Modified plank with chair**: Try small movements, bending your elbows slightly and lowering yourself toward the chair as if in a push-up. Repeat for 5 times.

- **Seated leg lifts**: Try holding your legs up for longer, keeping your stomach contracted. Do 10 repetitions, rest, then repeat for 10 more.

Day 6: Regenerative sequence with deeper twisting

On day 6, repeat the regenerative sequence, but focus on the twists. Try to hold each twist longer, for 7 breaths, and try to rotate a little more each time you exhale.

Day 7: Active rest and mindfulness

Even in the second week, keep your rest day active. You could try taking a walk outdoors, practicing *mindfulness* and focusing on the sounds and sensations around you.

These first two weeks help you solidify the basics and begin to make your practice slightly more challenging. Remember, every little bit of progress counts! The key is to be consistent and always listen to your body.

5.2 Week 3: Introduction of more advanced toning exercises

In the third week of your yoga program, we introduce slightly more advanced exercises to tone the body. These exercises will help you strengthen the muscles in your arms, legs, and core while also improving your posture. Don't worry, we will go step by step, and you will be able to adapt the exercises to your abilities. The important thing is to proceed slowly and not force your body.

Day 1-2: Core Toning

1. Plank with a chair (5 minutes)

Position: Start standing behind the chair, with hands resting on the backrest.

- Move your feet away from the chair so that your body is tilted, forming a straight line from your shoulders to your feet. Be sure to keep your body still and straight.

- Inhaling, bend your elbows slightly and lower your chest toward the chair, as if you were going to do a push-up.

- Exhale and return to the starting position. Repeat this movement 8-10 times.

- This exercise is more intense than the plank you were doing in previous weeks because it requires more strength in the arms and core.

2. Advanced leg lifts (5 minutes)

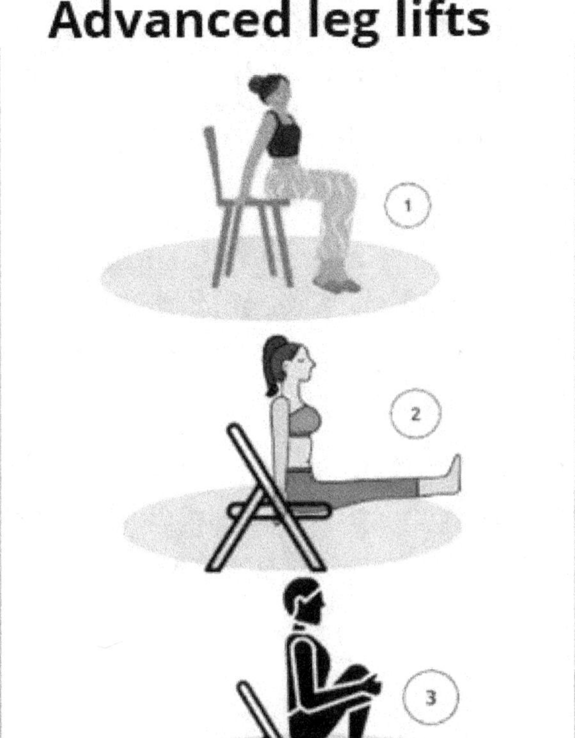

Position: Sit on the edge of the chair, with your hands resting at your sides.

- Inhaling, lift both legs together and bent, bringing them toward your chest. If you want an extra challenge, try lifting them outstretched.

- Hold the position for 2-3 deep breaths, then exhale and lower the legs slowly.

- Repeat for 10 times. If you feel tired, you can take a short break and then resume.

Day 3-4: Toning the Arms and Legs

1. Modified push-ups in the chair (5 minutes)

Position: As with the plank, stand behind the chair with your hands on the backrest.

- Inhaling, bend your elbows and lower your body toward the chair, keeping your body straight. Exhaling, push your body back to return to the starting position.

- Repeat this movement 8-12 times. You will feel the muscles in your arms and shoulders working harder than in the push-ups of previous weeks.

2. Chair lunges (5 minutes)

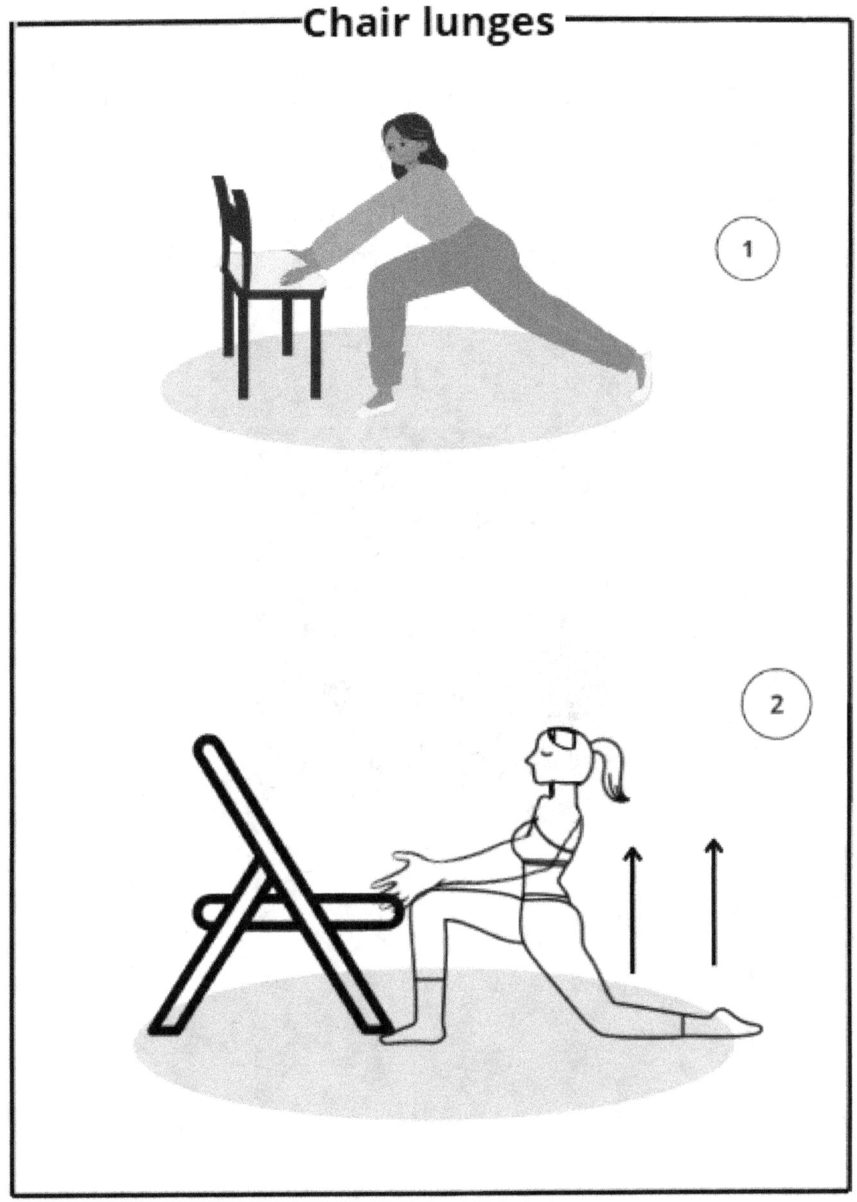

Position: Stand beside the chair and place your left hand on the backrest for balance.

- Inhaling, step back with the right leg, lowering into a lunge. The left leg remains bent at 90 degrees, while the right leg extends back.

- Exhale and return to standing, bringing the right leg forward.

- Repeat for 8-10 times on each side. This exercise helps tone the legs and buttocks, as well as improve balance.

Day 5-6: Complete Toning

1. Chair squat (5 minutes)

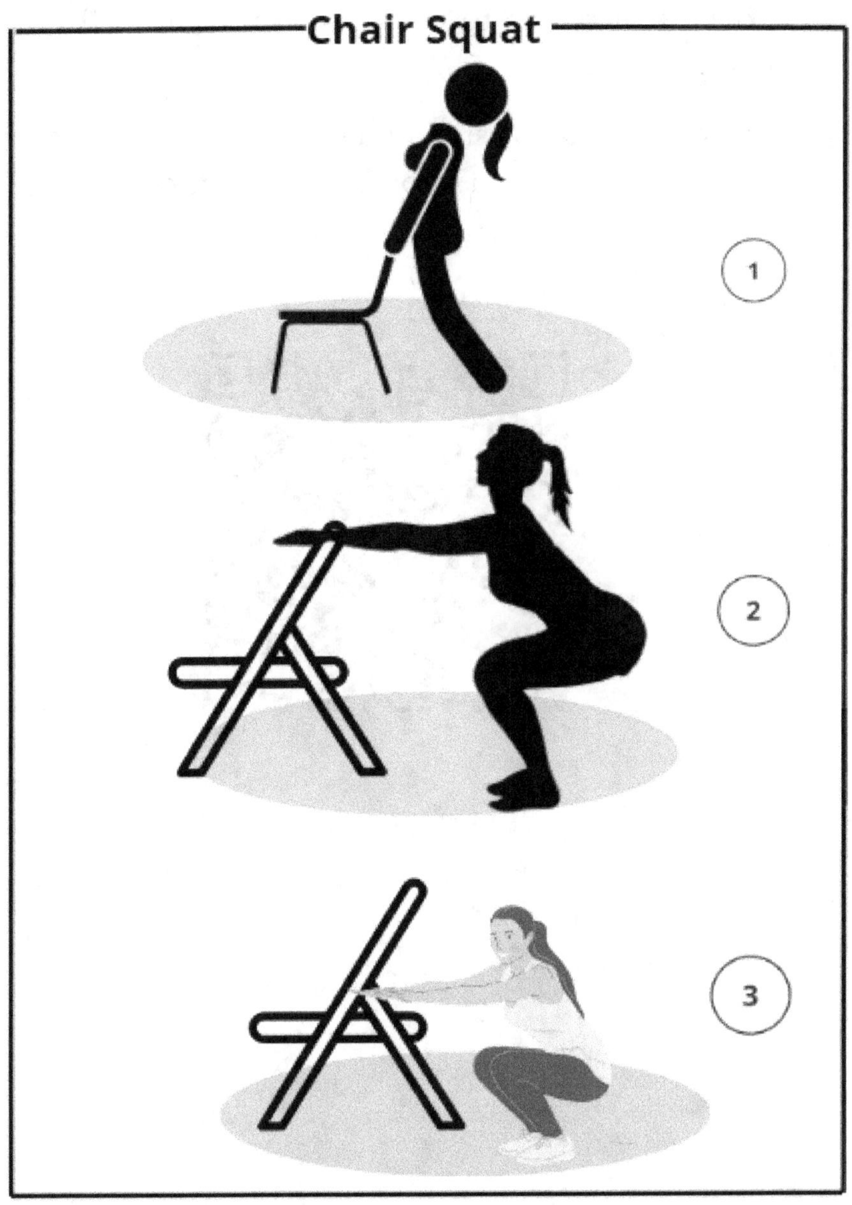

Position: Stand facing the chair, feet shoulder-width apart.

- Inhaling, bend your knees as if you were going to sit on the chair, but stop before you touch it. Keep your chest lifted and your weight on your heels.

- Exhale and return to standing. Repeat for 10 to 12 times.

- This exercise helps strengthen the legs and buttocks, and gives you an idea of how to perform a squat correctly.

2. Warrior II (5 minutes)

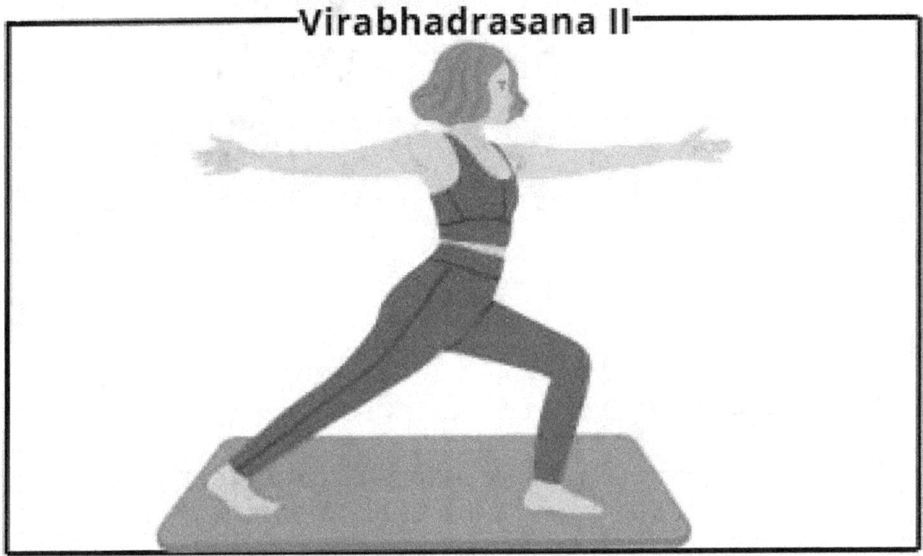

Position: Stand with feet apart. Turn to the right, bend your right leg to 90 degrees and extend your left leg back.

- Raise your arms parallel to the floor, one in front and one behind. Keep your shoulders relaxed and look over your right hand.

- Hold the position for 5 deep breaths, then repeat on the other side.

- This exercise tones the legs and arms while also improving balance.

Day 7: Active rest

On this day, you can take a light walk or do some stretching to keep your muscles relaxed and flexible. Rest is as important as exercises to allow the body to recover.

This week adds more challenging exercises to tone your whole body. In time, you will feel stronger and able to take on new challenges. Always remember to breathe deeply and move with awareness. Even if the exercises become more difficult, the important thing is to listen to your body and take breaks when you feel the need.

5.3 Week 4: Increase core and endurance intensity

In week 4, we start to make the *core* (abs and back) and resistance work a little more challenging. But don't worry, we will always go step by step and guide you step by step. The *core* is important because it helps you maintain balance and protect your back. Strengthening the core and increasing resistance will make you feel stronger and more confident in movement.

Day 1-2: Intensify the Work on the Core

   1. **Plank with movement (5 minutes)**

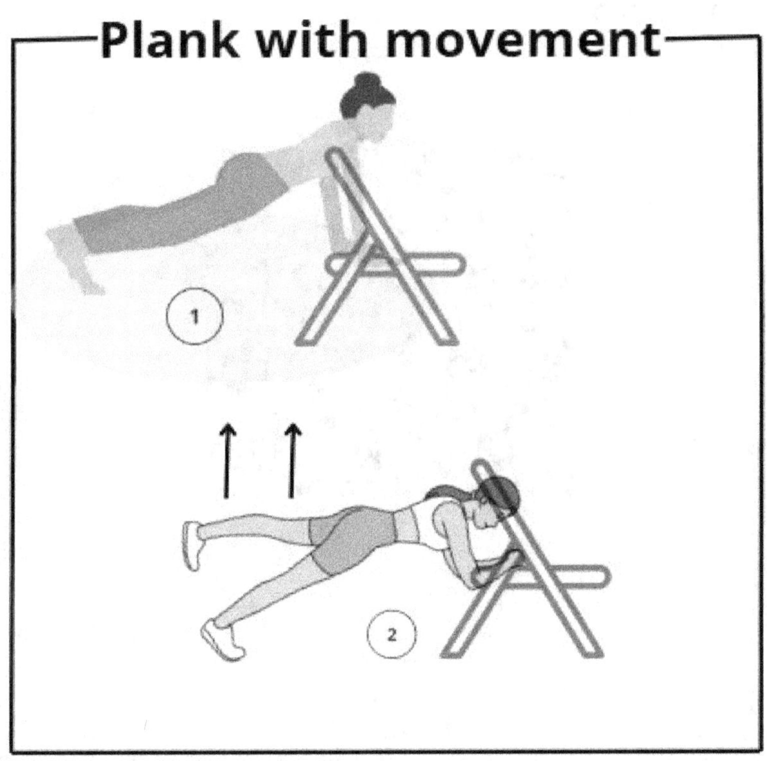

Position: Start standing behind the chair (or in front of the chair, depending on the type of chair available) with hands resting on the backrest.

- Move your feet away from the chair as for the plank, forming a straight line with your body.

- Inhaling, bend your elbows and lower slightly toward the chair. Exhaling, return to the starting position.

- After 3 repetitions, add a movement: raise one leg as you inhale, keeping it straight, then lower it as you exhale. Repeat alternating legs 8-10 times.

This exercise works the core and improves balance and endurance as you are combining movement with maintaining stability.

2. Bicycle sitting (5 minutes)

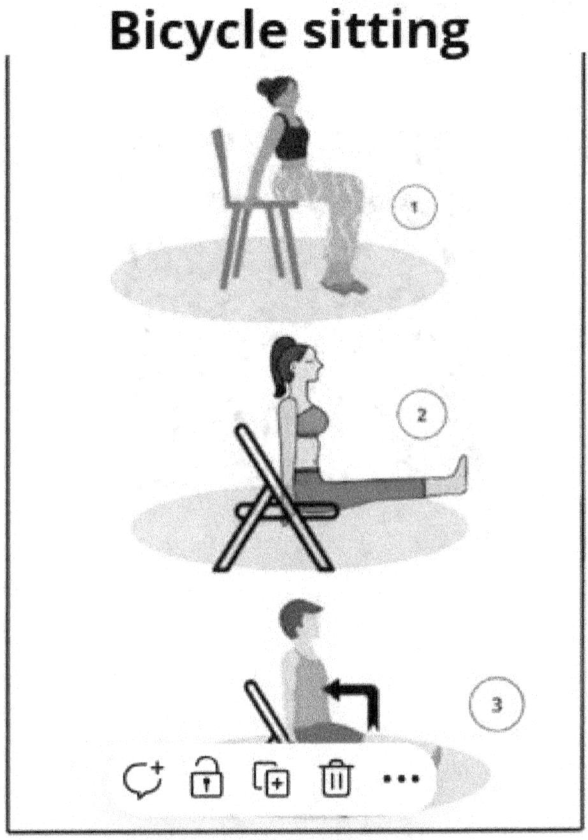

Position: Sit on the edge of the chair with your back straight and your hands on the sides of the chair.

- Lift both legs off the ground and bring your knees toward your chest. Now start moving your legs as if you were pedaling on a bicycle.

- As one leg approaches the chest, the other leg extends. Hold this movement for 10 repetitions, then take a short break and repeat.

This exercise is great for strengthening the abs and improving coordination.

Day 3-4: Resistance Work on Legs and Arms

1. Dynamic lunges (5 minutes)

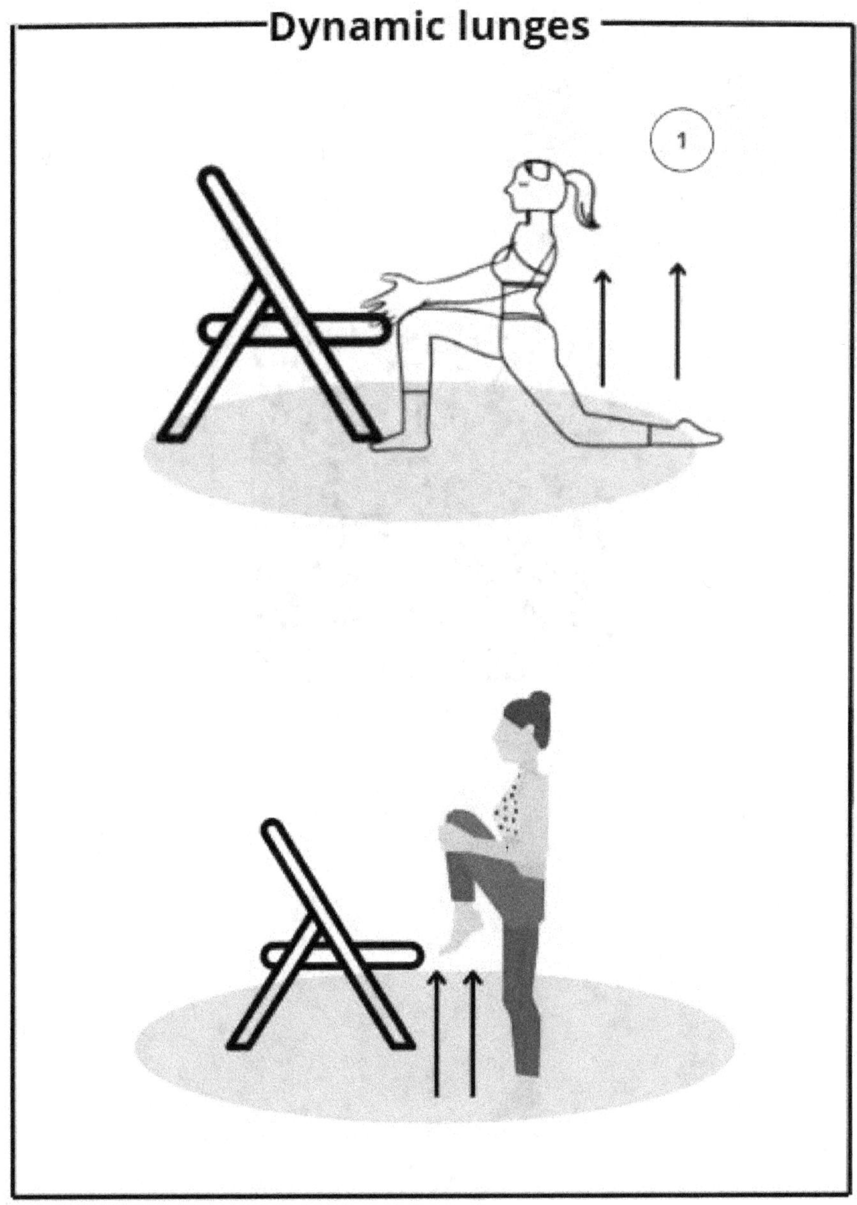

Position: Stand beside the chair, with your left hand resting on the backrest for balance.

- Inhaling, step back with your right leg, lowering yourself into a lunge. Exhaling, return to standing and bring your right knee toward your chest.

- Repeat 8-10 times on each side, alternating legs.

Adding the knee lift increases lunge intensity, improving leg strength and endurance.

2. Push-ups with chair (5 minutes)

Push-ups with chair

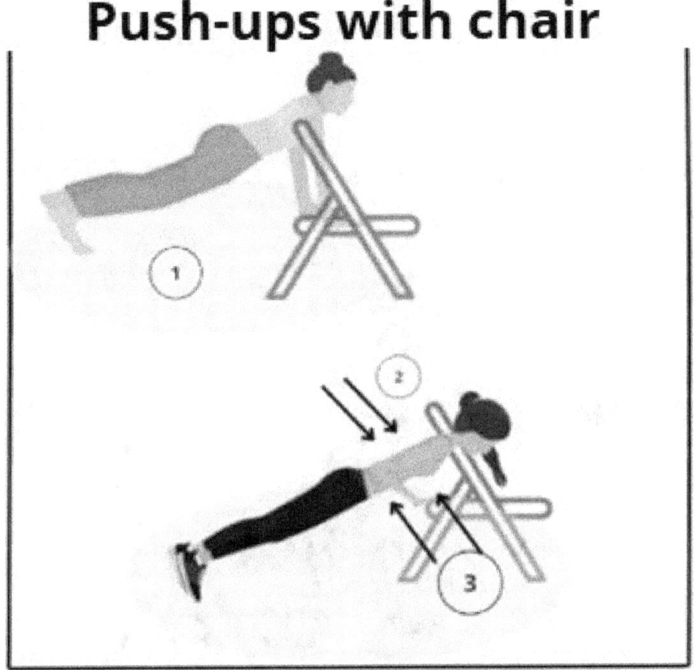

Position: As with the plank, stand behind the chair with your hands on the backrest.

- Inhaling, bend your elbows and lower yourself toward the chair. Keep your body straight and your arms strong. Exhaling, push your body back to return to starting position.

- Repeat for 10-12 times.

This exercise makes arms, shoulders and core stronger and improves endurance.

Day 5-6: Complete Resistance with Advanced Exercises

1. Dynamic squat with chair (5 minutes)

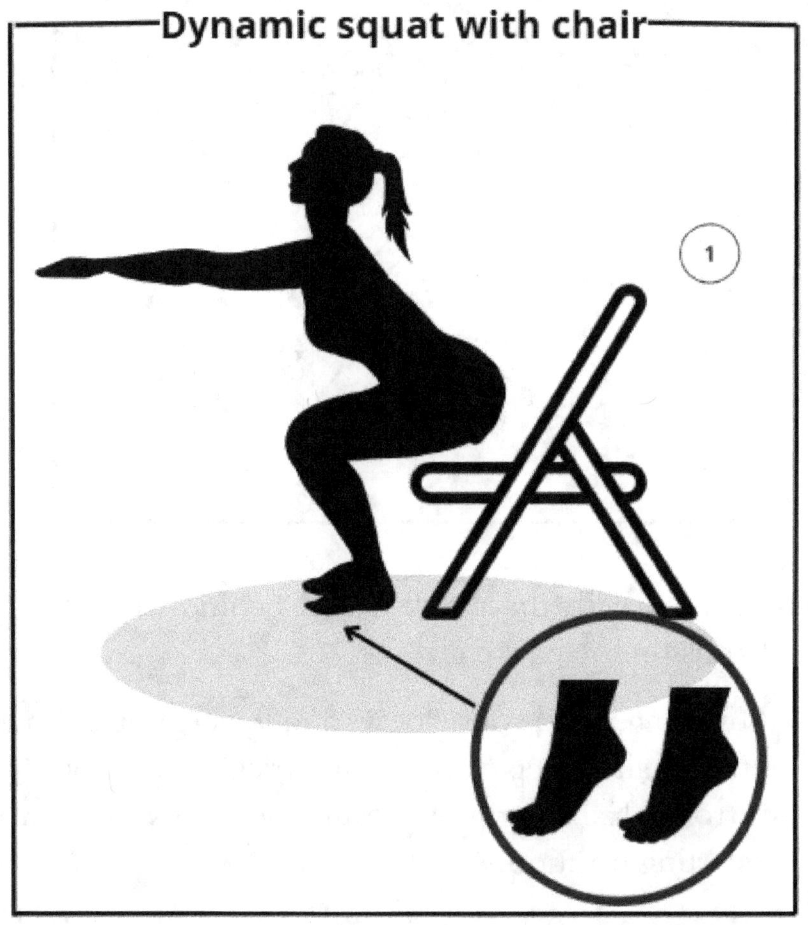

Position: Stand in front of the chair with your feet shoulder-width apart.

- Inhaling, bend your knees as if you were going to sit in the chair. When your legs are bent, instead of sitting down, lift yourself slightly onto your toes.

- Maintain balance for one second, then return to standing by exhaling. Repeat for 10 to 12 times.

This exercise strengthens legs and glutes and improves balance and endurance as you add the challenge of standing on your toes.

2. Position of the Warrior III (5 minutes)

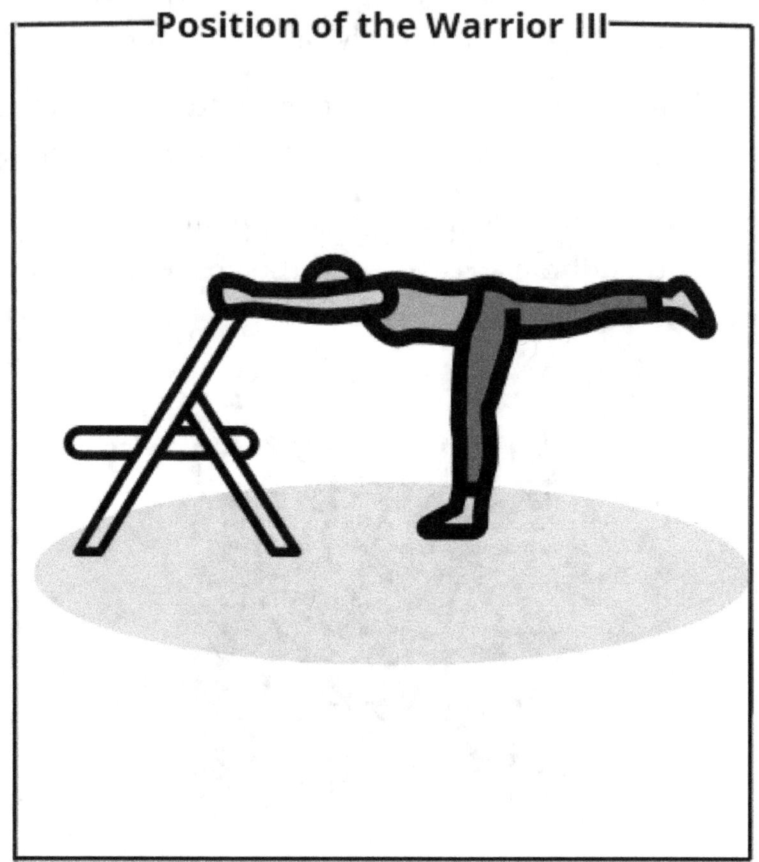

Position: Stand behind the chair with your hands resting on the backrest.

- Shift your weight to your left leg and lift your right leg back, keeping your body in a straight line, parallel to the floor.

- Raise your arms forward (you can hold them on the chair for support), keeping your balance. Hold the position for 5 deep breaths, then repeat on the other side.

This exercise increases core, leg and arm strength and improves balance.

Day 7: Active rest with deep breathing

After a busy week, take the day for active rest. You can take a light walk or devote a few minutes to deep breathing.

Breathing exercise:

- Sit comfortably in a chair or on a mat, close your eyes and breathe deeply.

- Inhale for 4 seconds, hold for 2, and exhale slowly for 6 seconds. Repeat for 5 minutes.

This week, you have increased the intensity of the exercises, working more on core, leg and arm strength. Keep it up and remember to do each movement carefully, breathing deeply to help your body stay strong and flexible!

5.4 Review week: Listen to your body and adjust the program

Review week is very important in your yoga journey. After a month of practice, it is time to stop and reflect on the signals your body is sending you. Yoga is not only about movement, but also about the ability to listen to what your body is communicating to you, both in terms of energy and any discomforts. In this week, I will guide you on how to interpret these signals and how to adapt the program to your needs.

Listening to Your Body

Your body speaks to you in many ways, and during yoga practice it is important to learn to listen to it. Here are some signs that may tell you to slow down or modify your exercises:

- **Sensation of pain**: If you feel sharp or persistent pain during or after practice, it may be a sign that you are pushing your body too hard. Yoga should never cause pain. If you feel pain, especially in joints such as your knees or back, it is important to stop immediately and reevaluate the exercise.

- **Overfatigue**: Feeling tired after an intense session is normal, but if you feel exhausted or fatigued in an unusual way, you may need to reduce the intensity of the positions. Extreme fatigue may be a sign that your body needs more rest to recover.

- **Shortness** of breath: Breathing is your ally in yoga practice. If you feel your breath becoming short or labored during the postures, it may be a sign that you are going beyond your limits. Remember to breathe deeply and adapt the rhythm of your practice to your breath.

How to Adapt the Program

Now that you have learned to recognize your body's signals, let's see how you can adapt the program to meet these needs.

1. Reduce the intensity of the positions

If you feel that some positions are too challenging, you can reduce their intensity. For example, if you find deep lunges or chair *plank* difficult, you can perform the easier variations:

- **Lunges**: Reduce the depth of the lunge by bending the back knee less.

- Plank: Keep planking for less time or avoid adding complex movements.

The important thing is that you feel you can maintain control over your body, without forcing your muscles or joints.

2. Increase relaxation sessions

If you feel the body needs more recovery, don't hesitate to add more moments of relaxation or meditation. You can replace a more intense session with a regenerative sequence, such as *Child's pose* or prolonged *Savasana*, to help the body relax completely.

- **Savasana**: Try extending the final relaxation for 10-15 minutes, focusing only on slow breathing and releasing all tension.

3. Take more breaks during practice

If you notice that you need more time to recover between positions, it is okay to take longer breaks. For example, between sets of lunges and squats, you can sit for a few minutes and take a few deep breaths. This will help you maintain energy throughout the practice.

4. Focus on positions that make you feel good

There will be some positions that make you feel stronger and others that may be uncomfortable. This is normal! This week, pay more attention to how your body reacts to different positions and focus on the ones that feel good. If a position bothers you, try changing it or replacing it with one you like better.

- **Example**: If you feel comfortable in *Warrior II* but find the *Tree Position* too challenging, try doing more repetitions of the *Warrior* and leaving the tree aside for a few days.

What to do if you feel good?

If, on the other hand, you feel the body responds well and you have energy, you can try increasing the intensity of the program slightly:

- **Hold the positions longer**: Try holding some positions for a few more breaths, feeling the muscles working harder.

- **Add a repetition**: If you're feeling strong, you can add an extra repetition to your favorite exercises, such as squats or chair push-ups.

Conclusion

The most important thing during this week is to listen carefully to your body and adapt the program to its needs. There is no right or wrong amount of exercise-you need to find the right balance between exertion and relaxation so that you get the maximum benefit from yoga without overloading your body. This will allow you to keep progressing with consistency and well-being!

5.5 How to maintain constancy in the long run

Maintaining consistency in yoga practice is one of the most common challenges. Even if you are enthusiastic and motivated at first, obstacles may emerge over time that make it difficult to continue. Therefore, it is important to build a mindset that helps you stay determined and not give up. Yoga is not just exercise, it is a path of personal growth, and in order to achieve lasting results, you need perseverance and patience.

1. Focus on the process, not the outcome

One of the secrets to maintaining consistency in yoga is to focus on the path and not just the results. If you focus only on the end goal, such as losing weight or becoming more flexible, it's easy to get discouraged when progress seems slow. Instead, learn to enjoy every single yoga session as a time to connect with your body and mind. Each day of practice is a small step forward, even if it seems like there is no immediate change.

- **Practical tip**: At the end of each session, take a minute to reflect on how you feel. Ask yourself, "Do I feel more relaxed? Has my body awakened?" Often the small benefits are only noticed when we take the time to listen to ourselves.

2. Create a regular routine

The key to maintaining consistency is to make yoga part of your daily routine, like brushing your teeth or eating breakfast. If you incorporate it as a habit, it will become easier to practice even on days when you feel less motivated. You don't need to do long sessions every day-even 10 to 15 minutes of yoga is enough to keep your practice alive.

- **Practical tip**: Choose a specific time of day to devote yourself to yoga, such as in the morning as soon as you wake up or at night before bedtime. Mark this time in your calendar, just like an appointment, and stick to it.

3. Set realistic and gradual goals

Having goals is important, but they must be realistic and attainable. If you set your expectations too high, you risk feeling overwhelmed and giving up. Instead, start with small goals, such as practicing yoga 3 times a week for 20 minutes, and gradually increase the frequency or duration.

- **Practical tip**: Each week, set a mini-goal, such as improving a position or increasing the length of a session. Achieving these small goals will give you satisfaction and keep you motivated.

4. Listen to your body

Yoga is not a competition, and it is not about achieving a perfect performance. It is important to always listen to your body and adapt your practice to your needs at the time. There will be days when you feel full of energy and others when you need to do lighter exercises or engage in relaxation. That's okay: what matters is to maintain the connection with your body, even on the most difficult days.

- **Practice tip**: If you feel tired or stressed, try a regenerative session with relaxing postures and deep breathing. You'll still be consistent in your practice, but you'll give your body the rest it needs.

5. Keep a positive and welcoming mindset

<u>**The right** *mindset*</u> for yoga is one of acceptance and kindness toward yourself. Don't judge yourself if you miss a practice one day or if a pose seems more difficult than usual. Yoga is a personal journey, and every day is different. Learn to be patient with yourself and celebrate your progress, big or small.

- **Practical tip**: Whenever you feel unmotivated, repeat to yourself phrases such as, "Every practice brings me closer to my well-being" or "I respect myself and listen to myself at all times." These positive affirmations will help you maintain a calm and motivated approach.

6. Find pleasure in practice

One of the best ways to maintain consistency is to find pleasure in what you do. If you view yoga as a time of well-being for yourself, you will be more inclined to continue. You can make your sessions special by creating a pleasant environment: light a candle, put on relaxing music, or practice in a place that makes you feel comfortable.

- **Practical tip**: Turn yoga into a wellness ritual. Before each session, take a few minutes to prepare the space in which to practice, making sure it is cozy and quiet. This will make the practice even more enjoyable.

Chapter 6: Advanced Positions for Core and Toning

6.1 Advanced Utkatasana for legs and core

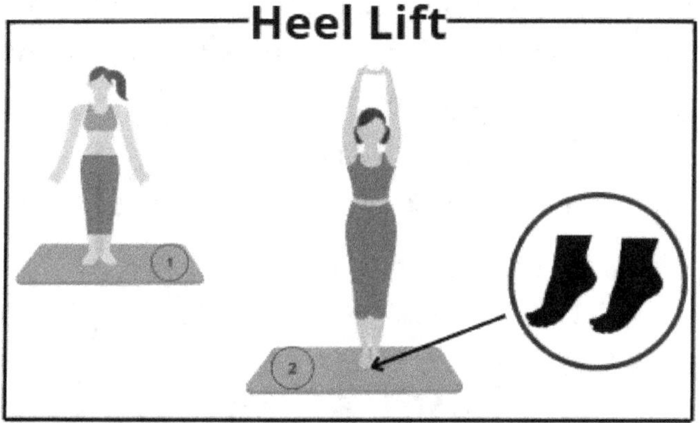

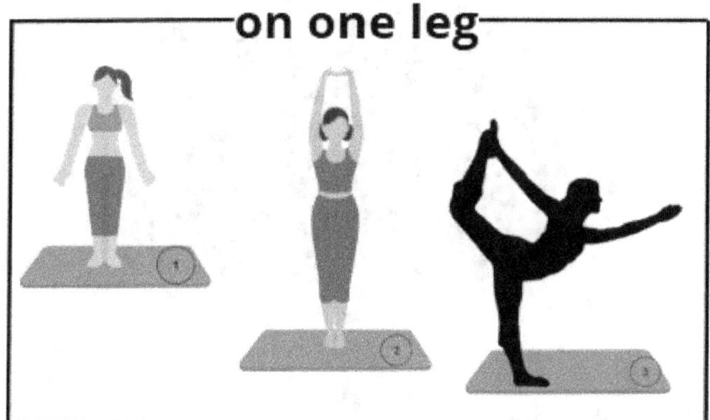

To make Utkatasana more challenging and intensify the leg and core work, you can try some advanced variations:

- **Heel** Lift: To add an extra challenge, try lifting your heels off the floor while in Utkatasana, keeping your weight on your toes. This requires more balance and intensely activates the core and leg muscles. Try to hold the position as long as possible without losing alignment.

- **Utkatasana on one leg**: Another advanced variation is to do Utkatasana by lifting one leg off the floor. You can start by lifting your left foot slightly off the floor and keep your balance on your right leg only, then switch sides. This exercise intensifies stability work and further strengthens the core and leg muscles.

Benefits of Utkatasana

- **Strength in the legs**: Utkatasana works intensively on the quadriceps, glutes and hip muscles, making it an excellent position for toning and strengthening the lower body.

- **Core activation**: Using the core to maintain balance and stability makes this position an excellent exercise for strengthening the abdominals and back.

- **Improves balance**: Advanced variations, such as heel lifts or single-leg holds, help develop balance and concentration.

6.2 Variants of yoga crunches for slimming

The abdominal variations in yoga are extremely effective in toning the abdomen and promoting weight loss. They work deep on the core muscles, helping to strengthen the abdominals and burn calories while improving stability and endurance. In this advanced exercise, I will guide you through a *Boat Pose* (Navasana) sequence and its variations to intensify core activation and promote slimming.

Exercise: Navasana (Boat Pose) and Variants for Slimming

1. **Starting Position - Preparation for Navasana** Sit on the mat with your legs stretched out in front of you. Keep your back straight and your core active,

lifting your chest slightly upward. Your hands can begin by resting behind your hips to give you support. From this position, while inhaling, bend your knees and lift your feet off the floor. Keep your knees bent at a 90-degree angle, with your shins parallel to the floor.

2. **Basic Boat Pose - Navasana** Once you have lifted your feet, try releasing your hands from the floor and extend them forward, parallel to the floor and facing your feet. Keep your torso slightly tilted back, but without arching your back. This is the basic Navasana pose, which intensely activates the abdominals. Breathe deeply and hold the position for 5-8 breaths, keeping the core active at all times.

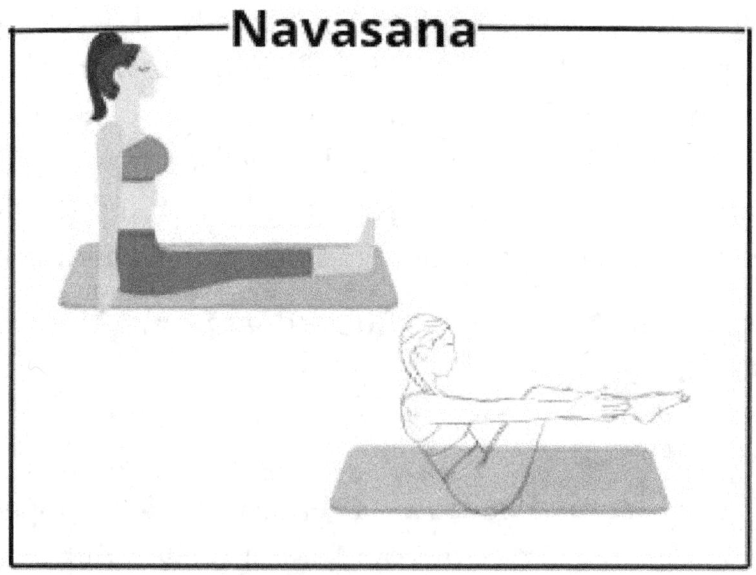

3. **Advanced Navasana - Leg Extension** To intensify the exercise, inhale and try to fully extend the legs forward, keeping them raised off the floor. This requires more activation of the core and legs. Keep your arms extended toward your feet at all times, and focus on maintaining balance and body control. Stay in this position for 5 breaths, keeping the focus on the core.

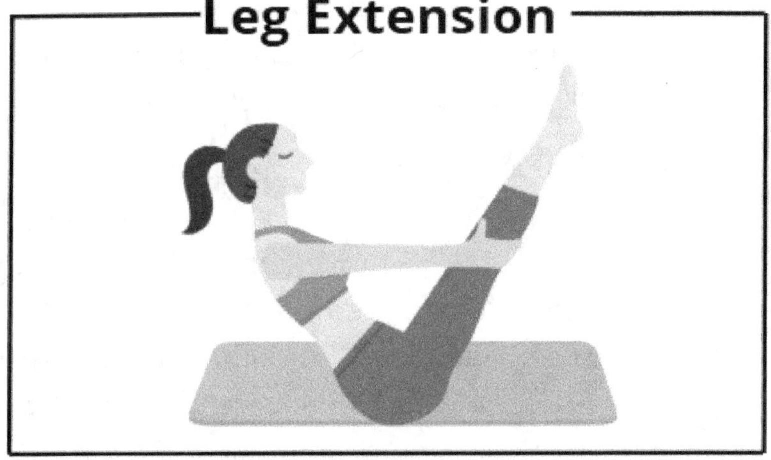

4. **Advanced variation - Leg alternation** If you want to increase the difficulty further and activate the oblique abdominals more, try leg alternation:

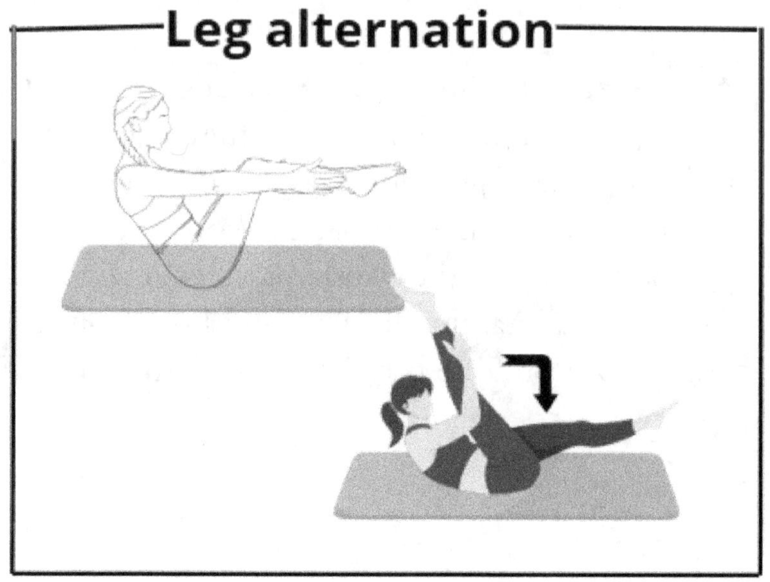

o Starting from the basic Navasana position with knees bent, inhale and extend the right leg forward, keeping the left leg bent.

o Exhaling, switch legs, extending the left and bending the right, as if you were doing a "pedaling" movement. Keep your arms extended forward and your torso tilted back. This dynamic movement intensifies the exercise and increases your heart rate, contributing to weight loss.

o Repeat alternating legs 10-12 times, always keeping the core active.

5. **Dynamic variation - Navasana with rotation** For an additional challenge, you can add a rotation to the torso:

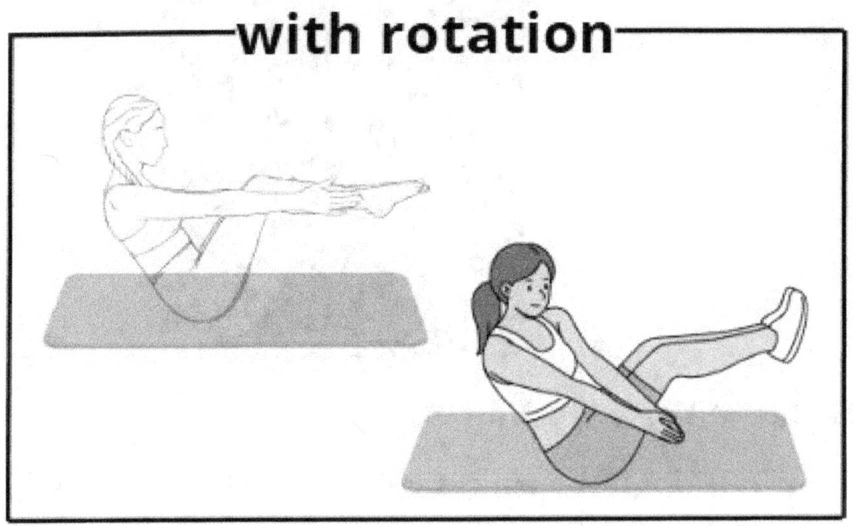

- o Starting in Navasana with knees bent, bring hands joined to chest in prayer position.

- o Inhaling, rotate the torso to the right, bringing the left elbow toward the outside of the right knee.

- o Exhaling, return to the center and repeat on the other side. This twist increases work on the obliques and helps tone the hips and lateral abdomen.

Benefits of Yoga Abs Variants

- **Slimming**: Dynamic variations such as alternating legs and twists increase heart rate, helping to burn calories and stimulate slimming.

- **Core strengthening**: These exercises work all the core muscles, including the deep abdominal bands and stabilizing muscles.

- **Improved stability**: Navasana and its variations improve body balance and stability, contributing to greater control in movements.

Chapter 7: Stretching and Relaxation Sequences for Recovery and Regeneration

7.1 Complete stretching sequence to relax shoulders and back

Relaxing the shoulders and back is essential after a day at work or an intense exercise session. A well-structured stretching sequence helps release accumulated tension, improve flexibility and promote muscle recovery. This sequence is designed to deeply stretch the muscles in your shoulders and back, allowing you to fully relax and rejuvenate. Follow the exercises step by step for maximum benefit.

How to perform the shoulder and back stretching sequence

1. **Starting Position - Sitting Comfortably** Start by sitting in a comfortable position on a chair or mat, with your back straight and feet firmly planted on the floor. Breathe in deeply and bring awareness to your posture, stretching your spine upward. Your shoulders should be relaxed and away from your ears.

2. **Shoulder Stretch - String of Pearls Position** Raise both arms above your head, interlocking the fingers of your hands. Inhaling, stretch your arms upward as far as possible, feeling the stretch all the way down your back and shoulders. Exhale slowly, lowering your shoulders and creating space between your ears and shoulders. Hold this position for 5 deep breaths, focusing on expanding the upper body.

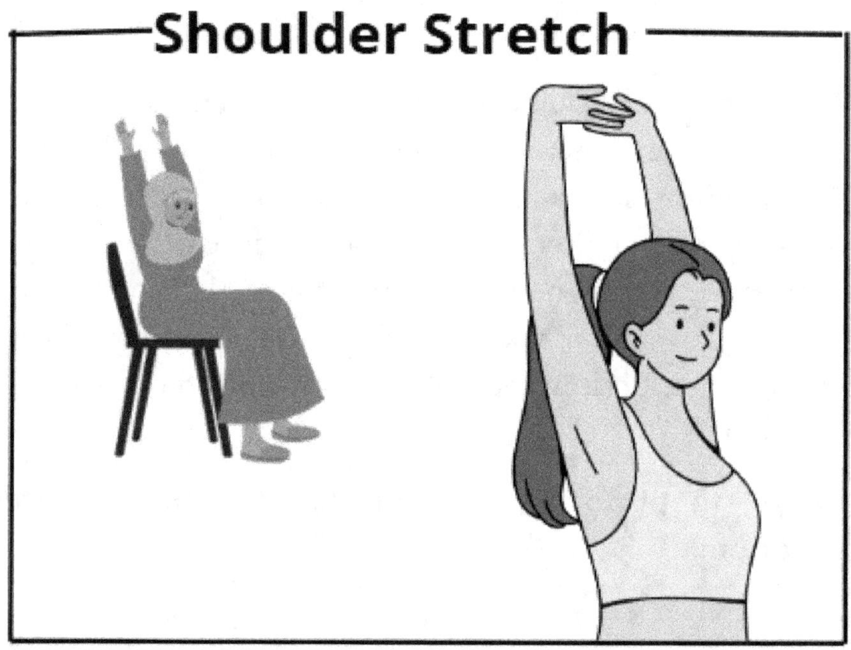

3. **Gentle back twist** Sit up straight and rest your right hand on your left knee. Bring your left hand behind you, resting it gently on the back of the chair or on the floor (if you are sitting on the floor). Inhaling, lengthen your spine. Exhaling, gently twist your torso

to the left, trying to look over your left shoulder. Hold the twist for 5 breaths, then return to center and repeat on the other side.

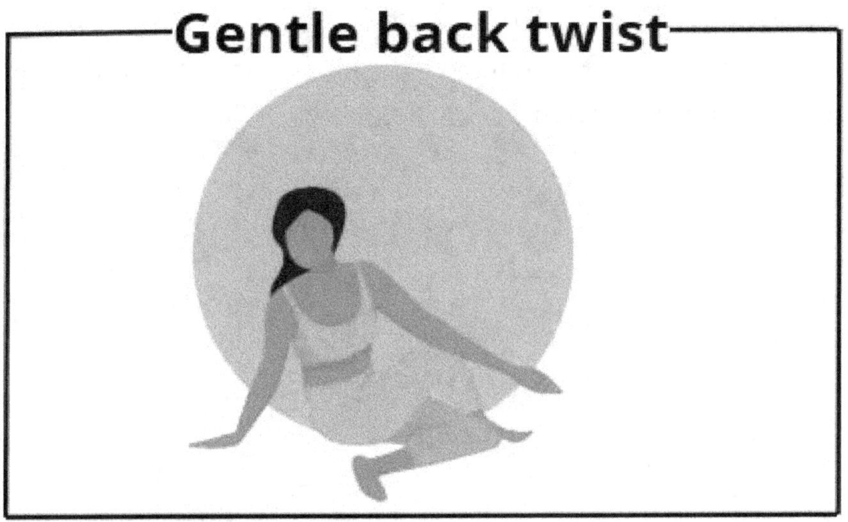

4. **Lateral Stretch - Shoulder Stretch** Lift your right arm upward and, inhaling, gently bend to the left, stretching the right side of your body. The left hand can rest on the side of the chair or on the mat for support. Hold the position for 5 deep breaths, feeling the stretch along the side of the body and shoulder. Return to the center and repeat on the opposite side, lifting the left arm.

5. **Forward back bend** Sit with feet hip-width apart. Inhaling, lengthen the spine. Exhaling, slowly bend forward from your hips, letting your torso relax toward your legs. Let your arms fall toward the floor or rest on your knees. Keep your head and neck relaxed. Stay in this position for 5-10 deep breaths, allowing your back to gently stretch and your shoulders to relax completely.

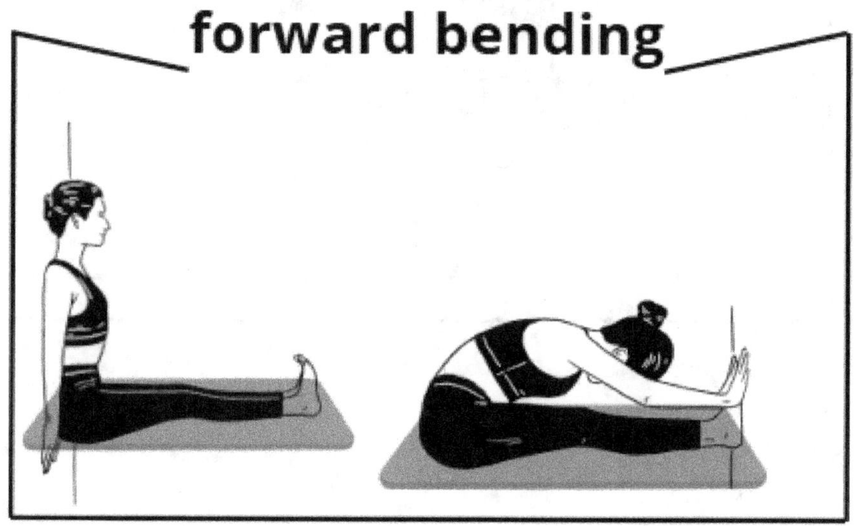

6. **Final Stretch - Modified Child's Position** If you are sitting in a chair, place your hands on the table in front of you and lean forward, letting your head come close to the tabletop. If you are on the mat, sit on your heels and bend forward, with your arms stretched out in front of you. Breathe deeply and relax for 5-10 breaths.

7.2 Forward bending and twisting to stretch the body

Forward bends and twists are two stretching techniques that deeply stretch the body, improving flexibility and promoting muscle relaxation. These movements are particularly useful for releasing tension in the back, hips, and shoulders, as well as stimulating circulation and improving mobility. In this sequence, I will guide you through a series of forward bends and twists different from those mentioned above, ideal for those seeking a more comprehensive practice to stretch the body.

Exercise 1: Forward Bend with Arm Extension

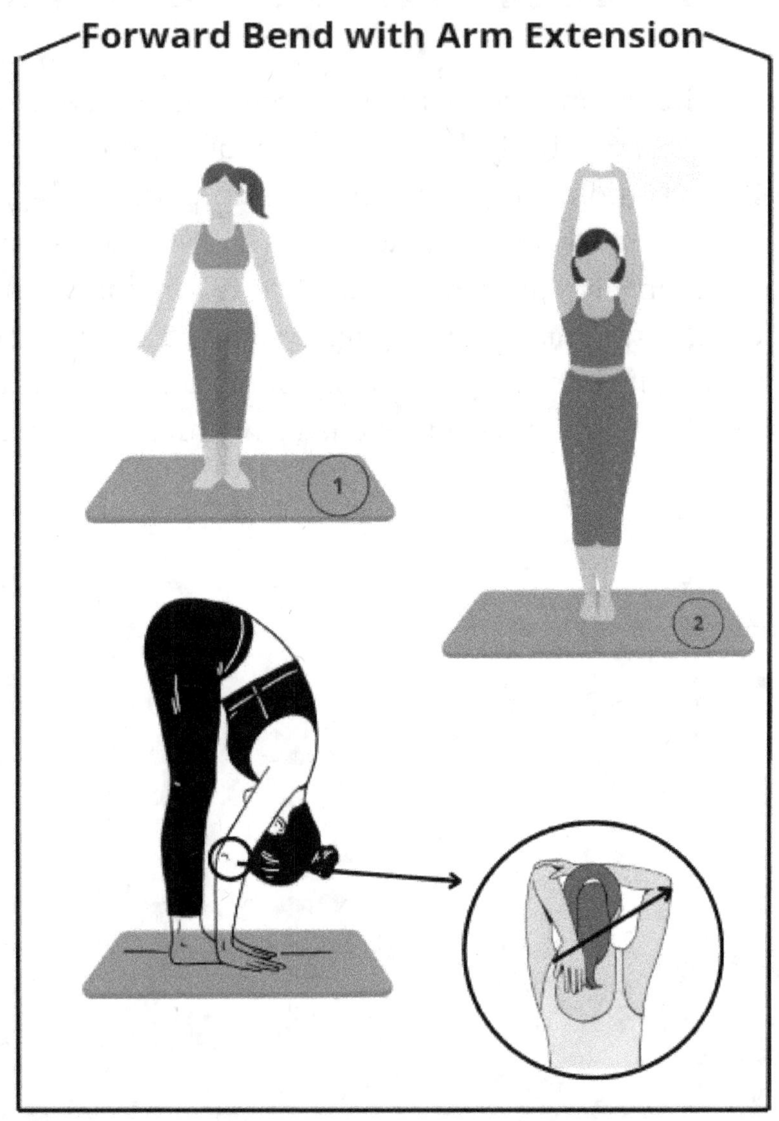

1. **Starting position**: Start standing, with feet hip-width apart. Knees should be slightly bent to avoid tension in the lower back.

2. **Forward** bend: Inhaling, stretch your arms above your head and, exhaling, slowly bend forward from your hips, keeping your back as straight as possible.

3. **Arm stretch**: Once bent forward, let your arms stretch toward the floor or, if you can, grab opposite elbows with your hands. This adds extra stretch to your shoulders and arms.

4. **Relaxation**: Let your head and neck relax completely, allowing gravity to do its work. Hold the position for 5-10 deep breaths. You can rock slightly from side to side to further release tension in the lower back.

Exercise 2: Cross-legged twist

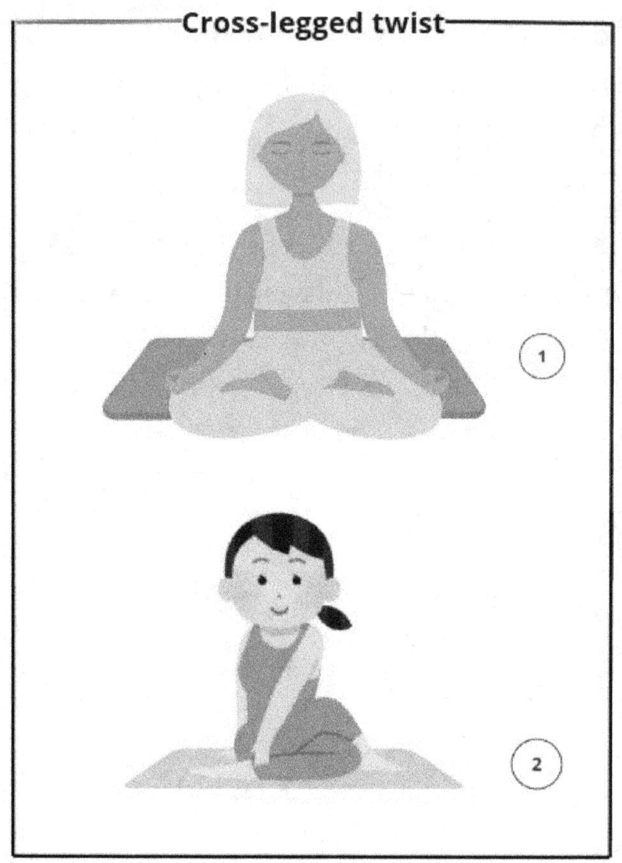

1. **Starting position:** Sit on the floor with legs crossed in a comfortable position, as in Sukhasana (easy pose). Keep your back straight and your core active.

2. **Begin the twist:** Inhaling, raise your right arm above your head, and exhaling, rotate your torso to the left, bringing your right hand to your left knee. Your left hand can rest gently on the floor behind you for support.

3. **Deepen the twist**: As you inhale, lengthen the spine upward. Exhaling, try to twist a little more, keeping your shoulders relaxed. Stay in the position for 5 breaths, then slowly return to the center and repeat on the other side.

4. **Advanced variation**: For more intense work, you can lift your torso while maintaining the twist, adding extra stretch to your hips and back muscles.

Exercise 3: Forward bend with legs apart (Prasarita Padottanasana)

1. **Starting position**: Stand with legs spread beyond shoulder width, keeping feet parallel to each other.

2. **Forward** bend: As you inhale, stretch your arms upward, and as you exhale, bend forward from your hips, letting your hands head toward the floor between your feet.

3. **Deep stretch**: If you can, bring your hands to the floor or grab your ankles for a deeper stretch. Keep your back straight and your core active.

4. **Relaxation**: Hold the position for 5-8 deep breaths, feeling the stretch in your hips, legs and back. For an advanced variation, try walking with your hands forward, stretching your back further.

<u>**7.3 Using deep breathing to reduce stress**</u>

Deep breathing is a simple but powerful technique to reduce stress and calm the mind. When we are under pressure or anxiety, our breathing tends to become shallow and rapid, which can increase physical and mental tension. Learning to use deep breathing can help you relax your nervous system and bring your body back into a calm state. Below we will explore some breathing techniques other than those commonly used in yoga to reduce stress and improve well-being.

Exercise 1: Diaphragmatic Breathing (Abdominal Breathing)

1. **Starting Position**: Lie on your back in a comfortable position with your legs slightly bent and your feet planted on the floor, or sit in a chair with your back straight and your feet resting on the floor. Place one hand on your abdomen and the other on your chest.

2. **Deep inhalation**: Inhaling slowly through the nose, concentrate your breathing in the lower abdomen. Try to expand the abdomen as if you were inflating a balloon, allowing the hand on the abdomen to rise. Keep your chest still, focusing solely on the movement of your abdomen.

3. **Long exhalation**: Exhale slowly through your mouth, drawing air completely out of your abdomen. The hand on your abdomen should lower as you exhale, helping you maintain focus on the breath. Repeat for 5-10 cycles of deep breathing.

Benefits: This deep breathing technique activates the diaphragm and slows the heart rate, promoting deep relaxation and reducing accumulated tension.

Exercise 2: Square Breathing (Box Breathing)

1. **Starting position**: Sit comfortably with your back straight, hands resting on your thighs and feet firmly planted on the floor. Close your eyes to better focus on your breath.

2. Inhale: Inhaling through your nose, count to 4 slowly. During this time, fill your lungs with air.

3. **Hold your breath**: Hold the air in your lungs for a count of 4. Don't force the holding, keep it comfortable.

4. Exhale: Exhale slowly through your nose or mouth for another 4 seconds, allowing the air to escape completely.

5. Pause: After exhaling, pause for 4 seconds before starting a new cycle.

Repeat for 5 to 8 cycles. This technique, also known as "box breathing," is especially useful for quickly reducing stress and calming the mind.

Exercise 3: Alternating nostril breathing (Nadi Shodhana)

1. **Starting position**: Sit comfortably with your back straight. Rest your left hand on your thigh and bring your right hand in front of your face, using your thumb to close your right nostril.

2. Inhale: Inhale deeply through the left nostril, keeping the right nostril closed.

3. **Switch sides**: Close the left nostril with the ring finger, open the right nostril and exhale through it.

4. **Inhale through the right nostril** and then close the right nostril again to exhale from the left.

Repeat for 5-10 cycles of alternating breathing. This technique helps balance the body's energy channels and calm the nervous system, promoting concentration and mental clarity.

7.4 Deep relaxation postures (e.g. Savasana, Supta Baddha Konasana)

Deep relaxation postures are essential to allow the body and mind to recover after an intense practice or stressful day. These postures promote muscle relaxation, deep breathing and mental calmness. Two classic postures such as *Savasana* (corpse pose) and *Supta Baddha Konasana* (supine butterfly pose) offer complete relaxation, but there are also other lesser-known variations that you can incorporate into your routine to achieve deep relaxation. Here we will look at two less traditional postures: *Viparita Karani* (wall leg pose) and modified *Balasana* with supports.

Exercise 1: Viparita Karani (Legs to the Wall Position)

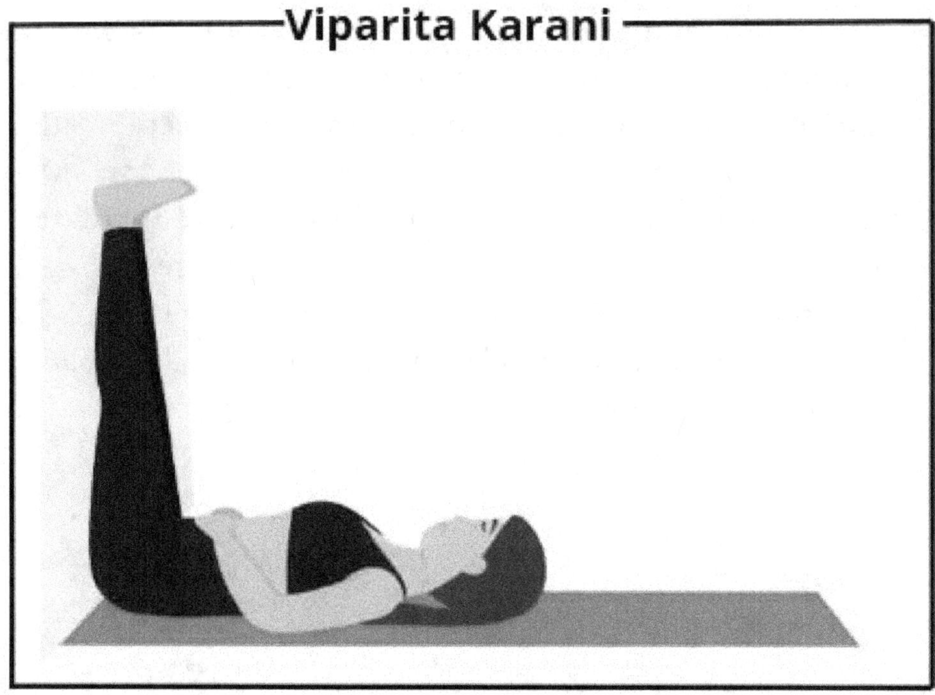

Viparita Karani is one of the best positions to promote deep relaxation, reduce leg fatigue and improve blood circulation.

1. **Positioning**: Lie on the floor with your buttocks as close to the wall as possible and your legs raised vertically, resting against the wall. Your arms can be extended along your sides, palms facing up, or you can bring your hands to your abdomen to feel the movement of your breath.

2. **Relaxation**: Close your eyes and focus on deep, regular breathing. Keep your legs completely relaxed, allowing gravity to do the work. If you want more

comfort, you can place a pillow or rolled blanket under your hips for a gentle lift. Stay in this position for 5-10 minutes.

Benefits: Viparita Karani promotes deep relaxation, helps reduce pressure in the legs and ankles, and stimulates blood circulation to the heart. It is especially indicated for those suffering from swelling or fatigue in the legs.

Exercise 2: Balasana (Child's pose) with Supports

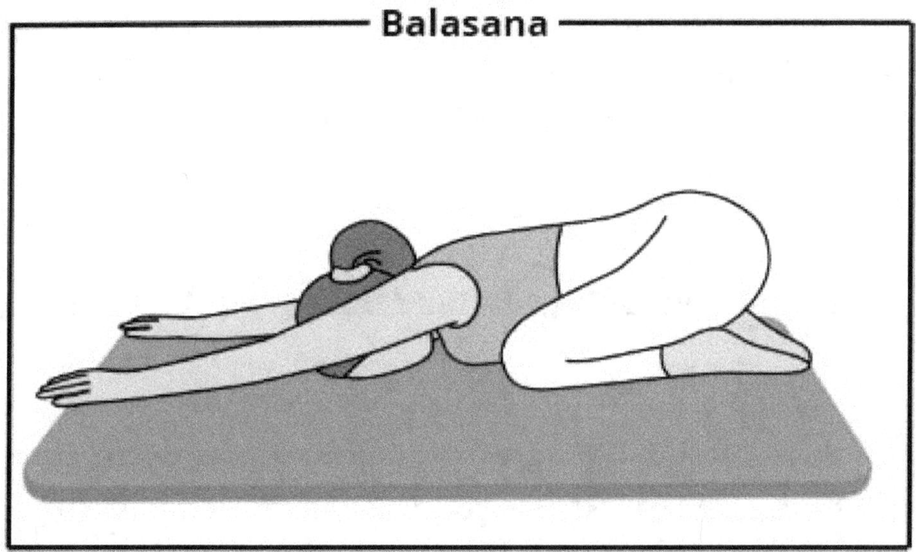

Balasana is one of the most calming postures in yoga, and when performed with the support of pillows or blankets, it becomes even more relaxing and rejuvenating for the body.

1. **Starting Position**: Begin by kneeling on the mat, with your knees slightly apart and your buttocks touching

your heels. Place a pillow or folded blanket in front of you, between your knees.

2. **Forward** bend: Exhaling, bend forward from the hips, resting the torso on the pillow or blanket. Arms may be extended forward or along the sides of the body, palms facing upward. The forehead can rest on the pillow or on a folded blanket for comfort.

3. **Relaxation**: Concentrate on deep breathing and allow the whole body to relax completely. Stay in the position for 5-10 minutes, allowing the muscles in your back, shoulders and neck to relax completely.

Benefits: Balasana with supports provides deep back and shoulder relaxation, and helps reduce stress and tension. The support under the torso allows you to hold the position longer without strain.

7.5 10-minute routine for the evening or after a busy day

Here is a 10-minute yoga routine for the evening or after a busy day. This sequence is designed to relax the body and calm the mind. Follow the steps given for each exercise, maintaining deep, regular breathing.

10-minute relaxation routine

FOR THE EVENING OR AFTER A BUSY DAY

	ACTIVITIES	TIME	PICTURE
1	**Child's Pose** Start by kneeling on the floor. Sit on your heels and extend your arms forward, resting your forehead on the mat.	2 Minutes	
2	**Seated Forward Bend** Sit with your legs stretched out in front of you. Inhaling, stretch your arms upward, and exhaling, bend forward to try to touch your feet.	2 Minutes	
3	**Reclined Pigeon Pose** Lie on your back, bring one ankle over the opposite knee and gently pull the leg toward you.	2 Minutes	
4	**Supine Spinal Twist** Lie on your back, bring your knees to your chest and drop your legs to one side, keeping your shoulders resting on the floor. Stretch your arms out in a cross.	2 Minutes	
5	**Legs Up the Wall** Lie on your back near a wall, lift your legs up against the wall and relax them. Keep your arms relaxed at your sides.	2 Minutes	

This routine is perfect for relaxing and recovering after a stressful day. Each position is designed to stretch and relax different parts of the body, promoting physical and mental recovery.

If you think you liked this book and it helped you, I only ask you to take a few seconds to leave a short review on Amazon!

Thank you,

Francesco Martini